**Praise for Kale**

"*Fantastic! One of the most entertaining health books I've ever read.*"

—Sara Gottfried, M.D., *New York Times* best-selling author of
*The Hormone Cure*

"*This is* The Omnivore's Dilemma *for anyone on a diet. This book takes you on a journey that explores why so much of what we think we know about diet is epically wrong—and then shares exactly what we need to do to really be healthy—how to eat right, feel energized, and never feel guilty about our food and lifestyle choices again.*"

—Nick Ortner, *New York Times* best-selling author of *The Tapping Solution*

"*Kale and Coffee isn't a typical health book—and that's a good thing. Think Michael Pollan meets Bill Bryson with a dash of Jon Stewart, and that will tell you how illuminating and enjoyable this book is to read. In fact, once I started I had a hard time putting it down. When was the last time you said that about a health book?*"

—Chris Kresser, *New York Times* best-selling author of
*Your Personal Paleo Code*

"*Kevin has graciously and articulately shared his ongoing health journey. His ability to sift through all types of health philosophies, protocols, and diets and come up with fresh, interesting conclusions—with a ton of humor and no bias—will help you determine what's going to improve your personal health. It's rare to read a health book that is both helpful and incredibly entertaining.*"

—Alan Christianson, NMD, *New York Times* best-selling author of
*The Adrenal Reset Diet*

# KALE AND COFFEE

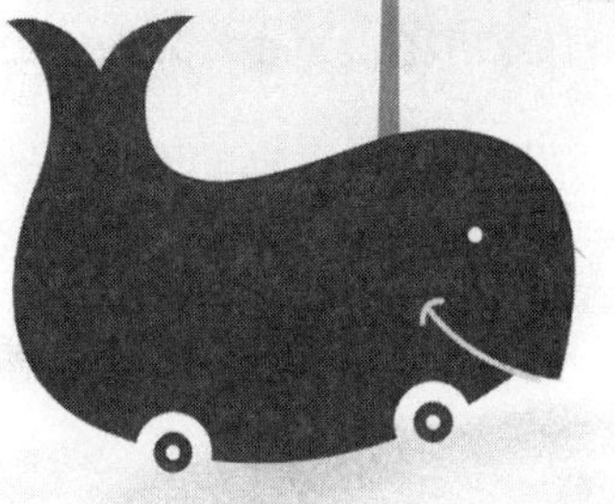

# ALSO BY KEVIN GIANNI

*The Busy Person's Fitness Solution: The Optimal Wellness System that Will Get You Motivated, Skyrocket Your Energy Levels, Boost Your Productivity, and Only Requires a Few Hours a Week!*

*High Raw: A Simple Approach to Health, Eating and Saving the Planet*

*Smoothie Recipes for Optimum Health*

Please visit:

Hay House USA: www.hayhouse.com®
Hay House Australia: www.hayhouse.com.au
Hay House UK: www.hayhouse.co.uk
Hay House India: www.hayhouse.co.in

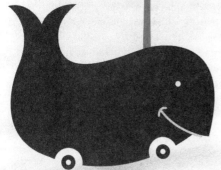

# KALE AND COFFEE

## A RENEGADE'S GUIDE TO HEALTH HAPPINESS & LONGEVITY

# KEVIN GIANNI

HAY HOUSE, INC.
Carlsbad, California • New York City
London • Sydney • Johannesburg
Vancouver • Hong Kong • New Delhi

*Published and distributed in the United States by:* Hay House, Inc.: www.hay-house.com® • *Published and distributed in Australia by:* Hay House Australia Pty. Ltd.: www.hayhouse.com.au • *Published and distributed in the United Kingdom by:* Hay House UK, Ltd.: www.hayhouse.co.uk • *Published and distributed in the Republic of South Africa by:* Hay House SA (Pty), Ltd.: info@hayhouse.co.za • *Distributed in Canada by:* Raincoast Books: www.raincoast.com • *Published in India by:* Hay House Publishers India: www.hayhouse.co.in

*Cover design:* Michelle Polizzi • *Interior design:* Riann Bender

**LIBRARY OF CONGRESS CATALOGING-IN-PUBLICATION DATA**

Gianni, Kevin M.
  Kale and coffee : a renegade's approach to guilt-free health, happiness, and longevity / by Kevin Gianni. -- 1st edition.
      pages cm
  ISBN 978-1-4019-4617-3 (hardback)
  1. Health. 2. Nutrition. I. Title.

  RA776.G483 2015
  613.2--dc23

**Hardcover ISBN: 978-1-4019-4617-3**

10  9  8  7  6  5  4  3  2
1st edition, July 2015

Printed in the United States of America

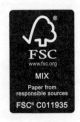
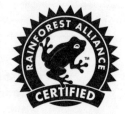

# CONTENTS

# INTRODUCTION

## BREAKING THE RULES

*"Never, never, never, never, never . . ."*

*Dave, the owner of Dave's RV, who has just installed tow bars on our SUV so we can attach our recently purchased motor home, pauses to take a breath. It is December 2008 and very cold in Connecticut.*

*On his exhale, his breath engulfs my wife, Annmarie, and me. He then continues, counting each word on his fingers till he reaches ten.*

*" . . . never, never, never, never, never back up."*

### Somewhere Outside of Pittsburgh, Two Weeks Later

Our new GPS has taken us on an unlikely route for an SUV. But we're in something much bigger: a 36-foot motor home with the SUV in tow. It's getting hairy.

A few minutes before, we turned off a four-lane road onto a residential street, then slowly climbed a steep hill. We have just descended, our engine brake gurgling loudly, and are waiting at a stop sign on the other side of the hill.

At the intersection, following our GPS instructions, I turn right onto a two-lane country road. Quickly, I see we might not make the turn, but it's too late to do anything else. I've already committed. We almost make it, but almost isn't enough. The RV nudges up against the guardrail on the opposite side of the road. We're now blocking both lanes of traffic.

Since we're stuck, now is probably a good time to start at the *real* beginning of this story.

It actually starts in bed. I know, it sounds racy—and it is, kind of—but not in the way you might think. Annmarie and I had just gotten into bed after a long day of work. She was a personal trainer at the time. I was also a personal trainer, but I was doing something a little more unusual for 2007. About a year earlier, I had decided to stop seeing regular clients and instead to produce daily health shows on YouTube. My mission was to change the world with a raw food diet, chlorella tablets, and life force. If that sounds crazy to you, you're not alone. I admit I was a little extreme back then.

Surprisingly, however, my plan was starting to work. Annmarie and I were both in the videos, and we had become big-fish-in-a-small-pond celebrities. Not the type who can't walk into a Walmart without being recognized, but the type who are regularly recognized in a health food co-op or Whole Foods Market.

But back to bed.

I mentioned to Annmarie that it was going to be a long haul of a career if we kept up the current grind. She was seeing clients all day, driving throughout southwestern Connecticut to get to them. I was sitting at a computer and filming my daily show with my Flip camera, hoping that one day we'd get a book deal, sell a million copies, and finally persuade all our family members to eat and exercise like us. Maybe we'd even move to the Hunza Valley, a Shangri La–like region in northern Pakistan, and live to be 150 years old together.

The reality was not as crystal clear. We were burning out. If we kept going at that pace, we'd eventually need our own personal trainers to kick our butts back into shape. On top of that, we were feeling unfulfilled. We had clients who were successfully following our programs, but we definitely were not having any luck with getting the family to eat healthy.

"What should we do next?" I asked Annmarie.

"Get an RV and travel around the country," she responded without a pause.

"Really?"

"Yep."

## Back to Our Little Unintended Road Block

Right now, I'm painfully aware of what that *yep* really meant and how much cozier it would be in our old bed back in Connecticut than in the driver's seat of this 30,000-pound beast.

I hear a horn honk.

My blood pressure is rising. We're blocking a road that has a surprising amount of traffic for before the morning rush. I want to throw our GPS out the window.

"What do we do?" Annmarie, always the water to my fire, asks calmly.

"I don't know. I think we have to back up."

"What about what Dave told . . . ?"

"Screw Dave."

I jump out of the driver's seat and open the RV door. At the back of the rig, I make a futile attempt to disengage the car from the tow bars. The angle of the RV and the weight of our car make it impossible. There's not even a millimeter of budge in the pins.

*Is this really how this trip going to be?* I mutter to myself.

Once we decided we were going to do a crazy thing like leave our families on the East Coast and hit the road indefinitely, it took only a few weeks to buy this motor home from a couple in Montana who had just crossed the country on their own sustainability tour. I had found them online, had emailed them late one night, and the next morning had woken up to a response saying they were putting their RV up for sale. Two days later, I saw a *New York Times* article about "green" RVs that the couple happened to be featured in. Annmarie and I believe in that synchronicity stuff, so we bought the RV. This was our sign that we were on the right path.

Less than 14 days after that, we were overnighting in a Walmart parking lot outside Cheyenne, Wyoming, in minus-15-degree weather. We had flown to Bozeman, Montana, the day before to pick up this surprisingly massive vehicle fueled by used vegetable oil.

With the personal training business scrapped and my Flip camera in hand—how's that for a business plan?—we were on the road. And with zero hours of RV driving under our belts, we were more dangerous than high-fructose corn syrup, trans fats, and heavy metals in tuna combined. Our mission was to learn as much as we could about health and nutrition, and upload it to YouTube. We were tired of having to dig deep to find answers about health. Our training clients, friends, and family members were coming up with some pretty interesting theories about health that made no sense at all. But they must have gotten them somewhere. We needed to find the people at the top of the misinformation chain and tie them up so they would never confuse anyone again. (Just kidding—kind of.)

## No Filming Here

On this slightly snowy, slightly cloudy day in Steeltown, there is no camera rolling.

I get back into the RV and sit in the driver's seat.

"Are you going to do it?" Annmarie asks.

"Yep."

I feel Dave's steaming breath cloud over my face again as she says this. He said "never" exactly ten times, one for each of his fingers. That's a lot of times. The dude was serious.

After the stern warning, Dave explained that when you back up a 36-foot Alpine Coach Motorhome with a Jeep Patriot attached to the stern, the Jeep starts to cut quickly at a serious angle. This doesn't really hurt the RV, but it wrecks the steering, shocks, and front axle of the car. And you can forget about the tow bars: they get mangled like blackberry brambles.

I ask Annmarie to get out, go to the back of the RV, and watch the car to see what happens.

"Stop me if you see or hear something," I tell her.

I put the RV into reverse, take my foot off the brake, then press the gas pedal lightly. The RV starts to creep backward. I realize that I've closed my eyes to avoid seeing whatever awful things might happen to the car or the rig, so I quickly open them again, but I can't see Annmarie in my rearview mirrors.

Another horn honks. The man in the silver Honda that is second in line to our left is starting to roll down his window. I assume it's only seconds before he shows me his southwestern Pennsylvania kindness in the form of a single-finger gesture.

"I can't see you!" I shout out of the side window. I know Annmarie can't hear me, but it's a way to vent my frustration.

I continue backing up, a few inches at a time, then put the RV into drive and whip the steering wheel in the other direction to gain a little more space in front. This turns into a four-point, then an eight-point, then a ten-point turn. The good news is that we're making progress. With seven more back-and-forth wiggles, I think we're good to go. Annmarie does, too. She rushes up to the front of the RV and checks the distance from the front of the rig to the guardrail.

"I think you're good!" she shouts.

I nod and wave her back inside.

With a deep breath of relief, I turn the wheel all the way to the right until it can't go any farther and step on the gas. We clear the guardrail, but through the open driver's-side window I hear a tearing sound. I know this isn't the car—if it were, it would be a more grizzly metal-on-metal sound—but there's no time to check what it is. *It can't be that bad,* I figure. We're finally moving, and we need to get to Kansas City to give a lecture for a hundred people in two days.


**A Few Hours Later . . .**

The last few hours of highway driving have helped reduce my anxiety about living in this vehicle for the next two or three years. We stop for lunch at an I-70 rest stop, and when I get out of the RV, I walk to the driver's-side front to check on the noise I heard before. At the bottom of the leather protective bib—the kind that keep big, flat-fronted vehicles like this from becoming bug collectors—there is a 12-by-12-inch hole. The guardrail had ripped the bib, and the torn material is now flapping in the cold air. *It's just a flesh wound, or maybe more of a battle scar,* I think. We didn't get out unscathed, but we're safe.

I get back in, and Annmarie hands me a bowl of salad. As we're eating, I wonder if Dave would have done the same thing we did.

Would he have broken the only rule he ever gives his tow-bar installation customers as they leave his RV repair shop? I think he would have. Sometimes when you're faced with strong evidence that what you're doing isn't working, it's time to go in a different direction. Sometimes you have to break the rules.

## This Book Is about Backing Up, Then Going Full Speed Ahead

When we left Connecticut back in 2008, we had a little bit of money and a YouTube following about as large as the city of Paducah, Kentucky, population (then) 25,577. But we had a dream and enough passion to be dangerous.

Over two and a half years on the road, we earned a master's degree's worth of experience while barreling down all the major interstates in our 36-foot classroom. We discovered facts about health and nutrition that neither of us could have imagined learning when we started out. We uncovered myths. We encountered health experts not practicing what they preached. We gave up our bodies for the sake of experiment.

During this time, people started paying attention. To this day, we've amassed over 10 million YouTube views and produced 932 shows. We get hundreds of thousands of visitors a month on our blog. I never did make it to big-league media like *Oprah*, but I was on the Kimora Lee Simmons reality show *Life in the Fab Lane.* Close enough.

But ultimately, the most shocking thing we found was that most of what we were doing in the name of great health was making us unhealthy. So we needed to rethink some things and back up a bit to get some clarity.

This book tracks our journey. I'll take you on a trip to the Andes and to a salt-mining operation in Mexico, a butchery class in California, and other places from which we culled important information. And I'll show you how to break the rules just enough, as we did, to get on the road to great health, great energy, and great lives. This journey is all about eating well, moving well, chilling out, and feeling amazing without having to give up the things you really, truly don't want to live without. This approach is guilt-free. Don't think kale, not coffee. Think kale *and* coffee.

While you're reading, you'll find some actionable tips you can implement right away. And at the end of the book, there's a 21-Day Jumpstart you can do if you want to throw yourself into transformation full force.

If you like, you can even skip to the Jumpstart right now, but if you do, you'll never find out why I gave up on almost everything I had learned about health and gained over 35 pounds in the year and a half after our RV trip ended.

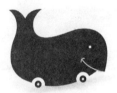

Our journey has included many more adventures than I could possibly cover in just one book. So if you feel like you want more, I encourage you to visit my websites, www .RenegadeHealth.com and www.KevinGianni.com. There, you'll find more insights, links to video interviews, photographs, and additional stories that didn't make the book but are extremely relevant to your personal longevity plan.

# CHAPTER 1

# FROM SKINNY, RAW FOOD VEGAN TO BLOATED, OUT-OF-SHAPE HEALTH BLOGGER

It's been almost six years since Pittsburgh, and I'm in front of my closet mirror with my pants half-buttoned.

I used to be in shape. I actually used to be one of the fittest guys in the room, but now I'm uncomfortable. I look bloated. I see the belly fat bunch together as I pull the button closer to the buttonhole. It doesn't make it. I don't want to leave the house today.

I check the tag of my Levi's 501s to see if by chance I grabbed Annmarie's. Nope. Size 34, and they're like sausage casing around my legs. I try one final time to suck in my stomach. It's not enough. The button won't make it.

You wouldn't think that a popular, sometimes publicly recognized health blogger with hundreds of thousands of people reading his work would dare to gain this much weight, but here is the proof that I had. I've become one of my personal training clients from years ago: uncomfortable, disgusted, self-conscious, asking Annmarie if I look fat just about every day. All in all, strange behavior for a guy who's never before thought twice about his weight.

What's harder to admit, though, is that I knew all along I was getting fatter, but I just ignored it. In fact, I didn't even care.

Four years ago, when I was something of a YouTube health celebrity, I was on top of the world. I also felt like I was on top of the diet pyramid. I ate the cleanest, most nutritious diet on the planet (or so I thought). A raw food, vegan diet. It was not only pure in its contents but also pure in its intention. With this type of diet, you eat straight from the earth, only as nature intended, never harming another living creature. I ate kale salad, raw nut butters, goji berries, raw chocolate, and dehydrated flax crackers. I drank green smoothies, green juice, wheatgrass, and hemp milk. I even tried a fruitarian diet, eating 3,000-plus calories of fruit every day. I tried all these different variations and more for four years. I guess you could say I was a little nuts about my diet.

The me looking in the mirror now would agree. All that health food made me neurotic. I thought about food from the moment I woke up to the second I fell asleep. While eating one meal, I'd be passionately consumed with what I would eat at the next. I was an addict in search of the purest dope: raw, vegan, organic food. When it wasn't there, I bitched, moaned, and jonesed, making me extremely unpleasant to be around.

I was headed down a path of self-destruction. So it's not surprising that, like any hard-core addict, I eventually hit rock bottom.

## Sick from Health Food

My extreme diet was so "healthy" that I made myself sick. About three years in, I started to notice that I was increasingly lethargic and was having trouble getting out of bed. In fact, I would wake up in the morning and stare at the ceiling, wondering if I was seriously ill: chronic fatigue, maybe, or multiple sclerosis, or cancer. After wondering for a while, I'd turn over and go back to sleep, not waking up again until 10 or 11 or even noon.

A few friends and family members suggested that the fatigue might be related to what I was eating, but I was so deeply indoctrinated in the cult of dietary purity that I wasn't willing to entertain their theories. It wasn't until I met a renaissance man of sorts, Dr. James E. Williams, that I listened to advice I didn't want to hear.

James is doctor of oriental medicine, board certified in naturopathic medicine, with a practice in Sarasota, Florida. He and I became close during the RV trip, and Annmarie and I spent time with him in Peru and at his home in Florida. James is the type of guy who can explain in fascinating detail how a viral infection can change your DNA, then follow with a story about dancing all night at a club in Havana, Cuba, while drinking brown rum and smoking local cigars.

I remember the day when he gave me the news that no vegan ever wants to hear: "Your adrenals are in deep fatigue. It's because of your diet. You might consider eating some animal protein"—meat, fish, fowl, dairy.

In the silence after he spoke, I imagined that I heard a cow's sad moo off in the distance. Another vegan was being coaxed off the wagon. But what James said wasn't just an opinion: he had tested dozens of my blood markers. Unlike my friends and family who had warned me about my vegan diet, James believed in science. He didn't advise on a hunch.

The numbers on half a dozen pages of lab reports didn't lie. As James ran through his own internal checklist, based on 30 years of practice, he read me in detail. I was shocked he could know so much about how I felt.

"I'm guessing you feel pretty lethargic, yes? Low sex drive? How about aggression? Do you have feelings of anxiety? Do you lash out with anger at things that you never did before?"

He nailed some two dozen more symptoms, but he only scratched the surface of what I was feeling emotionally. I was scared. My father died of brain cancer when I was two years old. My mother was diagnosed with breast cancer when I was just out of high school. She survived, but two out of two parents with cancer aren't great odds. You could say I got into this health thing because of what my parents went through. I wondered if feeling this way and continuing to eat this way would lead to a similar diagnosis.

What I had learned clearly wasn't working. All the lessons about superfoods, supplements, food combining, macronutrient balance, and more that I had picked up from numerous health gurus had produced the opposite results from what they were supposed to. Instead of being a superman, I had hormone levels lower than most men 50 years my senior. I wasn't working properly.

I also felt like a fake. Everything I had taught our blog readers and YouTube viewers had brought me here. Had they followed my advice, and were they feeling the same way? I was terrified that everything I had published on the Internet was ridiculously wrong.

So what did I do?

I did what any person would do who felt duped and scared after starting a diet he couldn't maintain. I quit. I quit raw food. I quit being a vegan. I gave up on everything. I de-stricted my diet and set myself free.

I figured that if all the information I had learned to date had produced unhealthy results, I might as well enjoy life, eating things that maybe weren't as nutritionally pure. I started eating whatever I wanted, but with a slight caveat. We live in California's East Bay—ground zero for America's farm-to-table movement—so I promised myself that I would remain on a 90 percent organic diet, since it is so easy here. From grass-fed beef to craft beer, from wine to French fries, I was now a consumer.

I laughed at portion sizes, ignored my lactose intolerance, and lived with my gluten insensitivity. I even got falling-down drunk—but only once. At first it was enjoyable—no, wait, it was awesome. I ate foods like scrapple (a mash-up of pork scraps, cornmeal, wheat flour, and spices), rillettes (meat pâté), and speck (smoked, cured ham)—things I never knew existed even before my raw food, vegan, and fruitarian experiments. I drank Pliny the Elder, possibly the highest-rated craft beer on the planet. I fell in love with sweetbreads. I would have mainlined Blue Bottle coffee if it were possible.

But as time passed, I started to feel that this probably wasn't going to end well either. My knees started to ache. I came down with more colds than I'd had in the past six years combined. I noticed my abs were getting soft. Some mornings depression crept over me like fog around the Bay Bridge, blanketing me in *can'ts, don'ts,* and *shouldn'ts*—doubts I'd never had before.

I was only one and a half years into this new regime, but I realized I was coming to the end of my run. Yes, it was a whole-food, organic diet, but it was almost as extreme as the one before—just in the opposite direction. I didn't want to stop, but I knew my health would suffer even more unless I did.

## The End of an Era of Extremes

Now, rummaging through my closet to find something that fits to wear to the office, I feel frustration. I push the hangers back and forth with waning hope that something that fits will appear. I wish that I could lose the weight tomorrow and have everything back to normal, but I realize this is impossible.

I manage to find a pair of hiking pants with an elastic waistband. I put them on with shame. I may have to wear them for two weeks straight.

On my walk to the office, I don't like seeing my reflection in the shop windows. I tell myself I can no longer ignore my present state. I tried to do so over the last 18 months, as I noticed my shirts getting tighter and my breath getting shorter as I walked up the two flights of stairs to our apartment. The detail that hit me hardest was the 9:20 mile I averaged in the inaugural Berkeley 10K race. Two years earlier, during a track workout, I had clocked a 6:22 mile.

When I get to the office, I decide to weigh myself on the UPS package scale. (We don't have a scale at home.) As I step on it, I feel like a cow being weighed before slaughter. The weight calculates slowly, reaching 223 pounds with clothes. I get off and on again. It's the same. This is the most I've ever weighed in my life. In 2011, at the height of my raw food experiment, I was 160. I admit, at 6 feet 2 inches, I looked underweight then. But today, in January 2014, about a year and a half after my anything-goes attitude swept me off my feet, I'm the complete opposite. I blew 38 pounds past my ideal weight of 185 in just 547 days. At this rate, 223 pounds isn't where I'm going to stop.

As I put away the scale meant to weigh our skin-care shipments, one of our team members opens the office front door.

"Weighing a package?" she asks.

"Yep," I say, as I slink out of the room. I look back to see her searching for the package.

## A Revolution Begins

It's at times like these, when I've been the most uncomfortable, that I've made incredible strides.

When we started our personal training business in 2005, we had no money. We thought Annmarie's network of physical therapists and athletic trainers would get us plenty of new clients, but none came. With only a few days to go before we missed a mortgage payment, we drove through the wealthiest neighborhood in town, placing flyers in the mailboxes of more than 400 homes. That brought us two clients the next day. One paid us up front in cash—the amount of our mortgage payment and more—and the other remained a client for the entire time we were trainers. Our unorthodox effort sparked our new careers then. Now is no different.

Determined, I promise myself this will be the first day of my personal revolution.

But I'm a reluctant revolutionary. I wish my diet of organic gluttony had worked. I wish I didn't weigh 223 pounds. I wish my cholesterol wasn't over 200 and my LDL-to-HDL ratio wasn't 2.8. I wish my omega 3 index was better than just average and that my pregnenolone hadn't dropped 34 points since the last time I was tested. (Pregnenolone is a hormone that's a precursor to other hormones, including progesterone.) I wish my jeans would fit. What I really want to be able to do is combine everything I've learned about health with the fun of eating whatever I wanted.

Isn't this the eternal health dream—to have our cake and eat it too? But I seriously wonder: can I take the best of both realms—a commitment to health and an anything-goes attitude—and find a way to live with them both? I am destined to find out.

I have already gathered much of the raw data. I have hundreds of expert interviews I've conducted, almost a thousand videos I've produced, and more than a thousand blog posts, many of them written from the road as Annmarie and I explored the United States in the RV, aptly named the Kale Whale by one of our readers. I also have all the health contacts I need to give me advice, answers, and tools.

This time, though, I promise myself that I'll examine everything through a different lens—a lens that looks for the details that matter most, not the screw-it attitude I had in the past. This time I want to keep only the techniques, foods, and diets that will bring the best results with the least effort.

You could say this is a renegade's approach. An approach that questions the gurus, the media, the companies that want you to buy their stuff. It's an approach that focuses on being smart, frugal, and knowing your body—something I'd given up on after that day in James's office. It's an approach that will require me to think outside the organic, farm-share veggie box.

I know deep down that great health does not need to be complicated. Now I intend to prove that to myself. So this is where I am: a bloated, out-of-shape health blogger with something to prove—to myself and also to you. I'm going to get back into shape on my own terms and show you that you can do it, too.

Up next, I'm at a swanky hotel in Beverly Hills, California, where I'm beginning to see why everything we think we know about health could be completely wrong . . .

# CHAPTER 2

# HOW *MY* 15 MINUTES OF FAME COULD SCREW UP *YOUR* QUEST FOR 90-PLUS YEARS OF LIFE

There are two television cameras facing me on the other side of the kitchen bar. Behind them at least a dozen people are buzzing around wires, microphones, and lights. But I'm the only person on the set, and I'm not the star. I'm getting nervous that this entire thing won't even happen.

Less than 48 hours ago, Annmarie and I were hiking to the top of Angel's Landing in Zion National Park in Utah. When we descended, I got a phone call from my assistant, Lisa. She had received a message from the Style Channel. They had seen our YouTube videos and wanted someone "hip and young" to put one of their reality stars on a juice cleanse.

Since there's almost no cell service in the canyon, we found a payphone and did a three-way call between the producer of the show, my team, and me. The program the producer was pitching is a reality show called *Life in the Fab Lane*. Kimora Lee Simmons is the star. I didn't know who she was, but I played it cool. The producer told me that she's a model and the CEO of a clothing line called Baby Phat. She's also the ex-wife of music mogul Russell Simmons. I was not getting booked on *Oprah,* but it was definitely a step beyond filming

YouTube videos on a pocket cam. I agreed to do the show. But there was a catch. The filming was in Los Angeles in less than two days.

With that, I hung up the phone, we headed to our car and drove out of the canyon to our RV. From there, we drove straight to California.

Now, 36 hours later, I'm in the same Beverly Hills hotel where the movie *Pretty Woman* was filmed, in a room that has been turned into a makeshift television studio.

## Waiting for Kimora

Kimora is over an hour late, and I'm standing next to a Tribest juicer, running my celery, carrot, and kale nutrition facts through my head. *Vitamin K for blood. One cup of kale has more vitamin C than an orange. Celery is a natural source of minerals.* I'm not as nervous as I thought I'd be, probably because it looks like the show may not happen at all. Also because, for reality TV, this is rather tame. No hot tubs, Long Island Iced Teas, or short skirts. I'm going to be teaching Kimora how to make a green juice—a juice of fresh vegetables and leafy greens—and I want it to be good.

This is my first foray into the health media guru game. *Dr. Oz must have started here, too,* I tell myself at the end of a mini pep talk. But, honestly, I'm wondering if it's even worth it. Am I really going to change the health of the world by showing Kimora Lee Simmons how to lose weight for a fashion shoot with a last-ditch juice fast?

Another 20 minutes pass and still no Kimora. The crew seems calm. They've set up the kitchen in this hotel room as if it were my kitchen at home. The idea is that when Kimora comes in, I'll be welcoming her into my apartment. An apartment that outside of reality TV costs $545 a day.

Ten more minutes pass. An intern comes back with more than a dozen bottles of Bolthouse Farms green juice. They want me to give Kimora a five-gallon plastic bottle of juice when it's time for her to leave. So we pour the bottled juice into the larger bottle. I'm starting to get the sense that it doesn't matter what happens during the taping—whether I make the juice or not, the final product will come out however they want it to. If Kimora doesn't show, they might even be able to tape us both at separate times and then edit us together as if we were in the same room.

Twenty-five more minutes, and finally the producer and co-producer come up to the kitchen bar. "Okay, Kimora is coming in now," the co-producer tells me. "Good luck. We'll be shouting suggestions for what to say from behind the camera."

Apparently, I am someone they know can be coached. Maybe I'm just a pawn—a guy with curly hair who fits the look they want. No wonder they asked me not to cut my hair before the taping.

Then the producer, maybe sensing my reservations, looks me in the eyes and says, "You'll be fine. You only have to remember one thing: reality TV is not reality."

What the producer said to me in that "studio" has echoed in my head ever since. If reality TV isn't reality, is it possible that the health advice we get isn't reality either?

The reason we're so confused about our own health is that the stories we've been told are a series of cuts, edits, and rewrites by the media, health gurus, companies, medical doctors, and researchers—in some cases, by total nutcases. And with all these fabrications, what has been lost is the essence of what great health really is and how to get it.


### Expert, Healer, or Nutcase?

Unfortunately, our modern health history is littered with stories of fraud, media mistakes, food company propaganda, slimy researchers, and lazy government regulation. The founder of Sensa, Dr. Alan Hirsch, tried to convince people that simply by tearing open a small pack of powder and sprinkling it on your food, you would see extra weight just fall off. What's more surprising than that fishy claim is that between 2007 and 2012, sales of Sensa totaled $364 million. Unfortunately, there's nothing in the ingredients—maltodextrin, tricalcium phosphate, silica, starches, fillers, and flavors—that could or would melt anything away except your bank account. It was no surprise that in January 2014, the Federal Trade Commission (FTC) cracked down on Sensa's marketing practices and imposed a $46.5 million judgment on the company.

Even Kellogg's ran afoul of the FTC in 2010[1] when it claimed that Rice Krispies "now helps support your child's immunity" with 25 percent of the daily requirement of antioxidants and nutrients—vitamins A, B, C, and E. The back of the box stated that the cereal "has been improved to include antioxidants and nutrients that your family needs to help them stay healthy."

The FTC said the immunity claim was not backed by scientific research. What's worse, the decision came just one year after the government organization cracked down on Kellogg's for making similar inadequately supported health claims about Frosted Mini-Wheats. The company stated that Mini-Wheats "improved kids' attentiveness by nearly 20 percent."[2] A 2009 settlement with the FTC banned Kellogg's from making claims about the cognitive benefits of cereals "unless the claims were true and substantiated."[3] With 21 percent of Frosted Mini-Wheats consisting of sugar, the only attentiveness increase I can imagine is that of the parent—who has to chase a sugar-fueled tornado all around the house.

Kellogg's is not the only manufacturer whose cereals have aroused concern. In a study assessing sugar content in children's cereal, 84 cereals were tested and the Environmental Working Group found that two-thirds of them were 24 to 26 percent sugar, and two cereals—Post Golden Crisp and Kellogg's Honey Smacks—surpassed the 50 percent mark.[4]

## Completely Tuning Out

Just as I examined how the media and corrupt companies operate as background for this book, I also did my research on Kimora before the taping. Thirty-six hours before the taping—actually 38, because she was 2 hours late—I bought *Fabulosity: What It Is and How to Get It*, Kimora's autobiography, and read it to learn more about her. The text wasn't as gaudy as the cover; it was actually motivating.

But the Kimora here in front of the camera is not radiating positivity. She's giving me a hard time. She's already answered her phone a few times during filming. "I don't want to do this," she announces.

I don't think she's acting, and I sense that her reality, beyond reality TV, is that she is worn out. If this is the case, I want to help her.

Finally, she says to the entire crew, "Come on, do I really have to do this?" There is silence on the set. I'm sure it doesn't go on as long I think, but no one speaks.

I decide this is my TV moment. Why not? Nothing is going as I thought it would, so I might as well step in. If she is, in fact, feeling miserable, then what I have to teach her will help. It will also help all the people who watch this show. Now is the time for me to inspire them to eat healthy. And so I take advantage of the opportunity.

I launch into the lamest personal development speech never to be heard on television. My "If you keep doing the same things, you'll get the same results," and "Where are you going to be if you keep living like this?" and finally my secret weapon, "In your book you say . . ." become digital pixels that will go straight to the editor's digital trash bin, never to be seen again.

When I'm done, there's more silence. No one on the set claps. There are no cheers. I don't even know if Kimora was looking at me when I was talking. After a few seconds of *what-the-hell-did-I-just-do?* I hear someone whisper, "We need to start wrapping this up." Then the producer breaks the silence and shouts, "Okay, Kevin, give her the juice."

This is my cue. Deflated but still obedient, I walk to the closet and grab the five-gallon bottle of fake juice. As I hand it to her, Kimora pretends to be shocked at its size. But she's not really shocked. She knew it was a ploy all along. I try to hold back a smile, since this is supposed to be serious. But this is not serious, not really. We're both actors putting on a show. She thanks me, and I walk her out my—I mean, the hotel room's—door.

## KIMORA LEE SIMMONS'S FABULOUS JUICE RECIPE

Here's the juice I prepared for Kimora Lee in the Tribest juicer on the set of her TV show:

2 to 3 large kale leaves
2 celery stalks
2 carrots
Handful of dandelion greens
½ cucumber
½ lemon
½-inch piece of fresh ginger (unpeeled)
½ green apple

## Back to Reality

A few months later, the show airs. Annmarie and I are watching it at a friend's house. As much as I wasn't nervous on the set, I'm anxious now. I don't know if they'll portray me as an expert or a kook.

On screen, Kimora comes to my "apartment." I'm portrayed as her "juice consultant," just one of the people on her team getting her in shape for her photo shoot. She's in "my" kitchen. We barely talk. I make the juice. They actually do a great job of making me look respectable. The maybe four-minute slot is seamless, and at the end I hand her the five-gallon bottle of the juice I didn't make, and she promises to drink it. That's it. My 15 minutes are actually 4.

This may be a good outcome. No one will get hurt, unless they make a five-gallon jug of juice and don't use their legs to lift it. But reality TV isn't reality. And my 15 minutes of fame won't make you sick, but misinterpretations of data, bad reporting, and deceptive marketing of food and health products most assuredly can.

Being on the *Life in the Fab Lane* set didn't launch my career as the next Dr. Phil, but it did reassure me that the only one in control of my own health is me. Same goes for you. Your health is too sacred to leave it up to the producers, the journalists, the gurus, the marketing directors, the researchers—even the agents of the FTC.

But where does this leave us? If we can't rely on the normal channels to tell us how to be healthy, where can we turn? Or, more specifically, as I'm often asked, *If I want to be healthy, what should I eat?* To find the answer, you and I have to go about things a little differently. No more TV, Internet, or guru worship.

So, don't be surprised that my exploration of this age-old question takes me to a beach in Costa Rica and an encounter with an unexpected thief.

# CHAPTER 3

# THE DUBIOUS DISTINCTION OF BEING THE ONLY ANIMAL ON THE PLANET THAT DOESN'T KNOW WHAT TO EAT

Annmarie and I walk out of the jungle and onto a beach in Manuel Antonio National Park, Costa Rica. It's hot, humid, and sunny, so we look for a place where there's enough shade to set up our little camp. We find a spot under a tree where the brush meets the sand and drop our gear.

It's May 2010. We're in Central America for, first, a friend's wedding; second, a five-day juice fast on the Nicoya Peninsula; and third, a three-day splurge at Tabacon, a natural volcanic hot spring. We've left the RV in Northern California. We're adventurous, but there's no way we were driving all the way down here.

After laying out our towels, we walk down to the water for a quick swim. The ocean is like bath water: warm and calm. But after just a few minutes, I feel the hot sun starting to burn my neck, and I retire to our towels for a nap. My 30-plus years as a very, very pale white man have taught me not to mess with the laws of UV radiation. I get 15 minutes max in the sun, so I choose it wisely.

I lie back, cradled in the sand under my towel, and close my eyes. This may be the first time I've relaxed in more than four years. It feels nice to let my thoughts go unfinished as I'm hypnotized by the gentle sound of the ocean lapping at the shore.

But somewhere between consciousness and sleep, my moment of bliss is interrupted. I hear an obnoxious chattering right behind me. Startled, but still groggy, I turn my head, and three feet away, next to our beach bag, is a raccoon. It's slimmer than American raccoons but clearly the same kind of scavenger. So far, it's managed to find our Ziploc bag of sliced cantaloupe and opened it up.

We look at each other for a moment. If the raccoon could speak, I'm sure he'd say, "¿Que mae pura vida?"—the laid-back Costa Rican way of saying, "What's up, dude?" along with their mantra of pure life. But I'm not as laid back as a Costa Rican raccoon. I want my food back. My first thought is to snatch it away from him. It is our only snack for the next few hours. He's messing with my blood sugar, which means he's messing with my marriage. That raccoon has no idea what a monster I can be if I don't eat.

I decide I can reach the bag without turning over and rehearse the plan of attack in my head as we stare each other down. But then another thought pops into my mind: the raccoon might have rabies. His mouth isn't foaming, and he doesn't look rabid, but I don't know anything about Central American rabies (or any rabies for that matter). I just know that getting rabies would really mess up the rest of our trip. I abort my plan.

The raccoon reaches into the open plastic bag, grabs a slice with two paws, and takes a bite. He's won. Then he runs off with the bag to eat the rest next to a tree a few yards away. I watch as he finishes the fruit and leaves the rinds.

What I don't know yet is that this is only the first invasion. Next, I hear clamoring from the jungle canopy above. Grunting, hooting, leaves rattling—this sound I know. Monkeys. And they're coming fast.

They swoop down from the tree, five of them, and run through the sand toward two girls who are sunbathing closer to the water. Their target is a shiny bag of what looks to be the Central American equivalent of Doritos. The girls don't have a chance to save their snack. One of the monkeys snatches it before they even see the thieves, and in a tornado of sand, all five of them retreat to the tree above me. They've done this before—their act is organized. They're pros.

The monkey who snatched the bag rips open the top, eats a few chips, then offers them to the others. The scene changes from a reconnaissance mission to a few dudes sitting around the TV, watching a football game. They cackle, eat, and wrestle as crumbs fall from above.

I have to admit, as much as I'm disappointed that I lost our snack, I'm amazed at how these animals operate. I'm sure this isn't the first time they've snagged a tourist's goodies. They're smart and resourceful. But as I watch the monkeys finish the chips, throw the bag to the ground empty, and hustle off into the jungle, I think about how weird it is to see monkeys eating Doritos.

There's nothing in a cheesy chip that even resembles what a monkey would normally eat. They don't each cheese. They don't eat corn. They don't eat vegetable oil. They don't eat salt. They don't eat MSG or artificial flavorings. What they do eat is fruit from the trees around them.

I realize that I've just witnessed two moments of dietary corruption. These monkeys and that raccoon live in one of the most visited tourist spots in Costa Rica. In a way, then, they're modern, adapted creatures. Because of the abundance of food on the beach and in the trash bins, or what people feed the animals despite numerous signs not to, the monkeys and raccoons have become domesticated enough to absorb some of the eating habits of the visitors.

They've become divergent—much as we have. But we're in much deeper than they will ever be. Our problem is that we've gone beyond opportunism, beyond snagging a bag of chips or a piece of fruit. We've made a foray into food creationism. We have managed to create foods and diets that have never before existed. Foods that are hybridized to have no seeds or to be dozens (if not hundreds) of times sweeter than their ancestors. Foods that are so stripped of nutrients that we have to add them back in. Foods that are genetically engineered—created by shooting the DNA of bacteria into their double helixes. Foods that can last in a box or can at the grocery store for longer than it takes to get a Ph.D.

What's worse—for our health at least—is that we eat these creations. No one's immune. It doesn't matter if you know nothing about health or you're a health freak. You eat some of them. I promise. For instance, a modern banana is not nearly the piece of fruit it used to be. It's been bred to be a supersized tube of sweetness, nothing like its smaller, starchier ancestors. Zookeepers at Paignton Zoo Environmental Park in England have stopped feeding bananas to their monkeys for this very reason. Amy Plowman, the zoo's Head of Conservation and Advocacy, likens our modern bananas to chocolate cake for monkeys, as we've bred most of the protein and fiber out of them, which is why they're causing gastrointestinal problems and even diabetes in the zoo's simian population.[1]

So here we are. We have no clue what our natural diet should be. Food—at least what we find in the grocery store—has changed so much, and the last few centuries of rampant dietary confusion (amplified in the last 50 or so years) have moved us further and further away from the real food we used to eat as a species.

## GMOS: FOODS NATURE NEVER DREAMED OF

Since the 1970s, food scientists have been tinkering with nature to produce fruits and vegetables that are disease-resistant, pack well for shipping, stay fresh longer, and have more shelf appeal. They've done this through genetic engineering—altering a plant's DNA by inserting genetic material from another organism. The result is a genetically modified organism (GMO). Corn and soy are two of the most common GMOs, frequently injected with bacteria that act as a natural pesticide. Corn and soy turn up as ingredients in literally hundreds of different processed foods. You won't find "GMO" on any label though. The Food and Drug Administration doesn't require it.

U.S. food safety experts claim there's no evidence that the GMOs on the market today are unsafe for your health. The rest of the world isn't so sure. A report by the Consumer Reports Food Safety and Sustainability Center states, "There is global scientific agreement that genetic engineering has the potential to introduce allergens and toxins in food crops, to change the nutritional value, and to create other unintended changes that may affect human health."[2] Animal studies in Europe have found evidence that engineered feed may adversely affect the liver, kidneys, gastrointestinal tract, and immune system.[3]

I, for one, don't want to eat tomatoes with fish genes inserted so they can stand the cold—or any of the many other Frankenstein-like foods. And I'm not alone: 72 percent of the people surveyed by *Consumer Reports* said they want to avoid GMOs when they shop, and 92 percent think engineered foods should be labeled as such. Not surprisingly, the food companies are vehemently opposed.

So how can you avoid GMOs? *Consumer Reports* suggest looking for products labeled organic or bearing the "Non-GMO Project Verified" seal. My advice? Don't eat processed foods, and you'll avoid the majority of genetically engineered foods. To avoid them altogether, buy farm-fresh produce grown locally.

For years, I've been researching how we moved so far away from our natural diets. We're the only animals on the planet who don't know what to eat. All wild animals know. Tigers don't eat kale. Wolves don't order superfoods from Tibet. Even Jonny 5, my domesticated cat, who is as wild as a slice of apple pie, has retained some of this knowledge. He won't eat Oreos or Cheez Doodles. Unlike most animals—even the monkeys from the beach, who I'm sure still eat foods from the jungle—we have completely lost the dietary wisdom of our ancestors.

My ancestors, at least some of them, are Italian. But my mom, grandparents, and extended family didn't teach me the ancient ways and recipes of our culture. My grandmother made us peanut butter cookies and snickerdoodles. I doubt the ancient Romans ate those treats. (But if they did they'd have been hooked; man, she could bake.)

It's a big deal that this knowledge is lost, because eating real food is the key to our survival as a species. If we don't figure out what foods we're supposed to eat—and how to eliminate the nonfoods we've created—we might wind up as an exhibit of bones in the extinct species wing of the American Museum of Natural History.

Even after all my own research, I still messed it up. I tried a few diets I thought were the ones I should be eating—not the diets of my ancestors, but ones I believed were more evolved and represent a philosophy of eating. The results were not good. The vegan diet— filled with plant proteins and no animal foods—messed with my hormones. I wanted it to work: it was noble to think I could eat healthy and barely harm another creature. The raw food diet didn't do what I wanted either, even though at the time I thought it was the most natural way to eat because it predates our species' use of fire. But both ways of eating were, for me, complete failures. And based on some of the evidence I'll present in the book, they're not really long-term solutions for anyone—for a human today, at any rate.

However, I'm an optimist, so even after my vegan and raw food experiments, I didn't stop searching. I wanted to find cultures (and researchers who were studying them) where people still know their natural way of eating and tend to live longer than others while eating these traditional foods. It's one thing to study cultures where people eat what their ancestors ate and live into their 40s, but it's another to find a few whose members routinely live into their 80s, 90s, and 100s. I was convinced that if I could find them, I could figure out definitively what I'm supposed to eat.

## A *Slight* Contrast, June 2011

I wake up in a panic. I can barely breathe. I'm confused. I don't know where I am, but I'm wrapped up tightly. I can't move my arms or legs. There's a loud rumbling, crashing sound outside. I wonder if this is death. *I'm young; this wasn't the plan; I'm not ready,* I hear myself say. Then I see gray canvas above me. I remember I'm in a tent.

But why? After a few more seconds, I snap out of my confusion. Annmarie is next to me. We're camping at 15,000 feet above sea level, at the base of Ausangate, a 21,000-foot peak in the Peruvian Andes.

This altitude is something I've never experienced before. The lack of oxygen has kept me in a half-awake daze all night, as have my stuffy nose and inability to catch my breath. Since sunset, the temperature has plummeted way below freezing, and I'm shivering. I'm in a zero-degree-rated sleeping bag, but I'm still cold, even though I'm wearing all the clothes I packed. Literally all of them—three pair of pants, four shirts, a sweatshirt, even two pairs of underwear.

I get out of my sleeping bag, unzip the tent, and go outside to find a place to relieve myself. It must be the middle of the night. The moon is bright. It lights up the snow-covered peak that towers over our camp. We're on the shore of a glacier lake that earlier in the day rippled whenever a breeze blew through. Now it's covered with a thin layer of ice. The crashing is the glacier speaking to us: grumbling, cracking, crumbling. I think it's letting us know it would like us to leave.

Besides Sebastian (our guide), Sebastian's friend, Annmarie, and me, there is no one within three hours' walking distance. This is by far the most remote place I've ever been.

As we ascended to our camp the day before, passing ancient stone homes with dried straw roofs, I realized that my quest to find our natural diet had taken me farther than I'd ever expected. I'd thought of going to remote places where people are still living the way they did thousands of years ago, but thinking about remote places and actually being there are quite different. We speak a little Spanish but no Quechua, the language spoken by Sebastian and his friend and most of the Q'ero villagers we passed on the way up. There's no cell service here and no place for an emergency helicopter to land. I'm scared out of my mind, but here I am, under the stars, with people from an ancient culture, observing what they do. My wish has been granted.

Almost. In some ways, Sebastian and his friend have been influenced by our modern lifestyles, although in others, they have not. Up here on this mountain, they're in their element. This is a spiritual place, a place to be revered. This trek is a snapshot of how they travel, how they lived until only a decade or so ago, when their environment as they had always known it began to change.

## A People Once Untouched

The Q'ero have lived in the Peruvian Andes for thousands and thousands of years. Some say they pre-date the Incans, others that they are descended from the Incans. To modern city folk in Peru they're simply Indians.

After the Spanish invasion, many of the Q'ero were pressed into service as slaves by the landowners on the haciendas—large tracts of land given to the conquistadors by the king for commercial activities like mining or farming. But where we are now—and even deeper in the Andes, where Sebastian is originally from—the haciendas ceased to exist a century or so ago because there wasn't much to farm or raise and there were no natural resources. As the Spanish abandoned the haciendas, they left the Q'ero with the land, the alpaca that roam on it, their Catholic names, and little else. The Q'ero have only recently come down from the mountains because there is no work and the climate is doing things it never did before. As James Williams explained it to me, the Q'ero believe that the natural cycle of seasons has been disrupted, compromising their ways of planting and harvesting, and threatening their survival. Now they're migrating away from a changed landscape into a new, more current one.

Before their migration into the cities and towns, the Q'ero ate a simple diet of potatoes, corn, alpaca meat, trout, and coca leaves. Coming from a health background, it was hard for me to understand how a diet with so little variety could be good for you. No foods from all colors of the rainbow. No spirulina. No Greek yogurt.

I had to see it for myself.

## A Conversation Best Left to an Interpreter

Two days before our trek to the glacier, I'm sitting with Sebastian at a table in his family's home in Tica Tica, an untouristy neighborhood of Cusco. Dense pockets of unfinished construction alternate with large tracts of eucalyptus forest. It's inhabited by not only the working class but also extremely unfriendly wild dogs.

We have just finished a meal of trout and potatoes that feels authentically Q'ero. We cooked the potatoes in a *watia*—a mini-igloo made of mud bricks, in which Sebastian burned branches and leaves to create coals. Once the *watia* was hot enough, we tossed in a few dozen potatoes and collapsed the mud bricks on top of them. Thirty minutes later, the perfectly cooked potatoes were ready to eat.

To round out the meal, we have a bottle of red wine I brought as a gift for Sebastian. He wants to drink it now, while we talk about the trek. It's 2 P.M., but I'm his guest, so I don't question whether this is a good time to drink. We have no bottle opener, so I tear off the plastic cover at the top of the bottle and push the cork down into the neck. Sebastian grabs a small wooden cup and motions for me to pour wine into it.

Then he smiles, dips his finger into the wine, removes it, and lets a drop fall to the ground. An offering to Pachamama—Mother Earth. Sebastian is not only Q'ero but a traditional Q'ero shaman. He's a community leader and healer, someone who communicates with the Apus, the mountain gods. He moved his family to Cusco out of necessity, to find work. A shaman is paid fairly well in Cusco because there are so many tourists looking for spiritual ceremonies. Having been in the city for over a decade, Sebastian lives in both worlds. It's evident in the way he dresses.

He wears a traditional Q'ero hat, a *ch'ulhu*, woven of alpaca wool with a rainbow-colored tuft hanging from each ear flap. His alpaca-wool poncho is also traditional, but underneath is a worn red-and-black North Face fleece. Around his neck is a pouch containing a bag of coca leaves—and a prepaid cell phone that rings every 30 or so minutes. Most of the calls are tour guides looking for Sebastian to come meet their groups.

It took only about three minutes of passing the wine bottle back and forth to empty it. I'm feeling pretty good, and my Spanish is more fluent.

"Vamos a Ausangate," Sebastian says in Spanish, inviting me to go to Ausangate.

"Sí. ¿Cuándo?" I ask him.

"Mañana."

"Okay," I say. "¿Cuántos dias?"

"No sé. ¿Cuatro?" he suggests.

"Sí, es posible. ¿Qué necesitamos?"

"Propane."

"Ok. ¿Algo más?"

"Tengo una carpa. Pero necesitas una bolsa para dormir."

"¿Hace frío?"

"No. No mucho."

If you don't speak Spanish, let me interpret. I have just agreed to take a four-day trek to one of the tallest peaks in South America with a tank of propane, a tent, two sleeping bags, a buzzed Q'ero shaman, and my wife. Oh, and he assured me it wouldn't be very cold.

I ask if we need an oxygen tank. He has no idea what I mean, but we both laugh anyway.

## Where Are the Potatoes?

The morning after my mini panic attack on the mountain, Annmarie and I find Sebastian sleeping outside by the ashes of the fire from the night before. His arms are tucked into his poncho. He has no blanket, no sleeping bag. I'm still wearing three pairs of pants.

I walk along the edge of the lake to explore and see where the food grows. We brought food with us on the back of a small horse, but I want to know where the people here would forage or grow food. But nothing grows here, not even moss or lichen. There's nothing but stone everywhere I look.

Even at 13,000 feet, where we camped the night before, near some Stone Age–looking homes, food was scarce. Any plant life was low to the ground, trimmed by the thousands of alpaca that roam the valley. I now understand why the traditional Q'ero diet appears so limited, with alpaca the preferred meat.

What I found, however, is that variety just comes in a different form: there are more than 400 types of potatoes in this region. Annmarie and I had already eaten at least 10 of them: red ones, purple ones, orange ones, starchy ones, and mushy ones, too. (If that sounds a little like Dr. Seuss, it should. Some of the potatoes look like they're straight out of one of his books.)

As for the rest of the Q'ero diet, it's largely seasonal. Corn, brought to the region from Mexico in the distant past, is grown at the lower elevations, where in the rainy season, the brown and barren landscape comes alive with all types of berries and edible greens. The Q'ero also dry their meat.

I look up at the mountain peak, jutting up into the cloudless blue sky. This is the top of the Q'ero world, and I'm sure living this high provided them protection over the centuries. No one could have survived up here without being as resourceful as they have been. They have learned to grow crops at a multitude of elevations up and down the mountains, while taking advantage of the seasonal abundance of other fresh foods. They've domesticated quinoa and amaranth, and hybridized potatoes for flavor and size. Coca leaves, which are nutritious as well as sacred, grow almost two miles closer to sea level than where we are now.

In short, the Q'ero have more variety than I thought, but they also eat the same staples over and over again. It's a relatively simple diet and to someone from Northern California, relatively boring. Was it possible that this entire trek—with the cold, the thin air, the fear of being so far away from civilization—was going to conclude with the revelation that we have to start importing Peruvian potatoes, chewing coca leaves, and hanging alpaca carcasses in our home to dry? Not exactly.

The first challenge to adopting the Q'ero diet is genetic. I'm not Q'ero. My background is European. I may or may not be able to thrive on potatoes. It would be foolish to assume that just by observing the Q'ero and how they live and eat, I would gain a diet blueprint for all people, including me, to follow.

The second challenge is that the Q'ero aren't documented as being as long-lived as some other cultures, even though anecdotally, they are considered so. It would make more sense, then, to study and possibly adopt the diet of those with the greatest confirmed longevity, right?

Well, kind of.

In 2004, journalist Dan Buettner set out with *National Geographic* to study the world's last existing long-lived cultures. After identifying a handful and verifying their ages, Buettner began to scientifically deconstruct what these cultures did, with the aim of creating a formula anyone could use to help reclaim their health and add as much as 12 quality years to their lives. His work, documented in the book *The Blue Zones*, may be some of the most convincing longevity research ever done.[4]

The five cultures—the Sardinians in southern Italy; the Nicoyans in Costa Rica; the Seventh-Day Adventists in Loma Linda, California; the Okinawans in Japan; and the natives of Ikaria in Greece—have the greatest number of people living past 100 years in the world. So it's only logical to think that if you want to live a long and healthy life, you should ask people who are doing it already and follow their lead.

But if you're looking for answers on what specific foods you should eat, you'll be disappointed, just like I was. The findings Buettner uncovered are generalities, not specifics. One of the main reasons is that the five cultures don't eat the same foods. There is no single, universal longevity diet or food. Just like the Q'ero, each Blue-Zone culture eats foods that are native to its land or were brought in through trade many generations before.

Additionally, many of the people in these cultures don't even eat foods we consider health foods. They don't eat chlorella—chlorophyll-rich algae popular in many health food circles (also known to make your teeth green for hours). They don't all eat egg whites for breakfast or toasted gluten-free bread. They eat what's available and in season. The amount of variety in their diets differs as well.

The Nicoyans, for instance, eat a staple diet of beans, corn, and squash, and that's pretty much it. But their longevity, even compared to other Costa Ricans, is evident. According to Buettner their rate of cancer deaths is 23 percent lower than the rest of the country's.

For many years, the Okinawans of Japan subsisted almost entirely on a diet of sweet potatoes, getting 80 percent of their calories from this one source. It seems that both Okinawans and Q'ero thrive on potatoes. But even if I were to decide, based on the evidence of these two longer-lived cultures, that my healthy diet required potatoes, how would I choose between the 400-plus varieties of the Andes and the one or two varieties from Japan?

The lack of culinary crossover between the longest-lived communities and the all-over-the-map amount of variety in their diets leads me—and Buettner—to conclude that the question *What are we supposed to eat to live long?* can't be answered with a list of specific foods. There is no one diet for longevity; in fact, in the Blue Zones, there are five. So how do you choose?

The only conclusion I can fully stand by looks at what *not* to eat. Longevity is more about what you leave out of your diet than what you include.

One of the major dietary factors the Blue Zone cultures share is that they don't eat excessively hybridized foods, genetically engineered foods, fast food, packaged foods, foods grown in mineral-depleted soils, animals injected with antibiotics and hormones, or any other category of food our modern world has created. But even at this level of simplification, there is a problem. Adhering to the what-you-leave-out rule doesn't give you permission to eat any organic foods you want without repercussions. Remember my 38-pound weight gain? Just because the Weston A. Price organization—a non-profit committed to restoring nutrient-dense foods to our diets—says raw butter is good for you, it doesn't mean that you can replace your morning tea with a cup of hot steaming butter.

So we need to use a little caution. We're supposed to eat freshly grown foods from our region and eat more plants than foods from any other food group. And whatever we eat, we're not supposed to overdo it. It's like Michael Pollan's quasi-haiku from his bestselling book *In Defense of Food:* "Eat food. Mostly plants. Not too much."[5] None of the Blue Zone diets includes meat as a staple, although most of the people eat it occasionally. What's also clear, however, is that they don't need to megadose with nutritionally dense superfoods, as many modern experts suggest. The foods grown in their natural soils contain enough minerals. Everyone gets enough protein from their diet. Everyone gets enough vitamin C. Everyone gets the right amount of iron.

James Williams clarifies some of the similarities in the Blue Zone diets with his own summary of the research: "All the consistently long-lived people are mostly coastal or mountainous, and all have fish in their diet. They all are high plant-based eaters, so there's lots of fiber. They also eat seasonally. I think another component is that they each have what we call superfoods. Whether they are seaweeds, as in Okinawa, or small amounts of wild honey, super-foods are a factor."

"Finally," James continues, "there is always some type of highly concentrated polyphenol, meaning an antioxidant. The Andean people have coca leaves. The Chinese have green tea, the Nicoyans the coffee bean, and the people of the Mayan Riviera, cacao or chocolate."

So if you want to live long like someone from one of these cultures, your diet needs to contain lots of plants, maybe some fish, a superfood or two, and a polyphenol-rich food or drink. And a ton of things need to be left out.

What a boring conclusion. It's so basic. I almost feel duped. I was taught that a healthy diet is so much more than it really needs to be. And I actually suffered because of what I learned. But I promise I'm not going to cop out on you with this lame conclusion. There really *is* more to it.

## Back to the Mountain

Sebastian is cooking a piece of alpaca in a skillet. The burner is fueled by the propane he told us to bring. There are about three cups of oil in the small pan, and it's splattering everywhere. The propane and the frying oil are definitely not traditional. And the fact that the oil is threatening to spill over with the slightest tilt of the pan makes this situation a little dangerous.

Once the meat is finished cooking, we share it, tearing off pieces with our hands, then passing it around. It tastes gamey, but it's good. After we finish, a teenager dressed in traditional Q'ero garb appears from farther down the mountain. In one hand he has a woven sack about the size of a backpack. In the other, a radio. He had to have hiked at least three hours to get here.

After a few minutes of chatting with Sebastian, he smiles at Annmarie and me and opens the sack. There are two 22-ounce bottles of Cusqueña, a beer brewed in Cusco. He's brought the party. After some coaxing, I agree to pay a few *soles*—Peruvian currency—for one, and he opens it. The beer is warm, but after the last few days,

I feel like this will be good medicine. The teen turns on the radio. The music bounces, as a nasal female voice sings in Quechua. Sebastian asks if we want to learn how to dance.

All five of us take turns—sometimes alone, sometimes in groups, stomping around a circle defined by our fire pit. The laughter and repetitive beat of the songs are trance inducing, and I find myself getting lost in my thoughts.

This is the simple life. Simple eating. Simple living.

It works for the Q'ero, but will this simple prescription work for me? Physically, it's clear I'm not one of them. I stand more than a foot taller than any Q'ero I've met. My genes are different.

One of the principles of longevity that Buettner and James Williams speak of is the long-established connection between culture, genes, and food. The Q'ero genes have adapted to the foods they eat over thousands of years. Unfortunately for me, I'm not from the same lineage that they are, or from any other long-lived culture. I'm a mutt. I'm in large part Italian—though there's no Sardinian in the mix—and also part Irish, part English, and part Polish, to name a few. The only connection between culture and food in my family is their false premise that pasta is a superfood that effectively boosts athletic performance and pacifies family dysfunction. It is also the embodiment of pure, motherly love.

And what about my health-food friends who are equally scattered genetically? Or the ones who are eating a simple longevity diet but are sick? Or the people who have adverse reactions to certain foods included in the Blue Zone diets? Why can some people drink milk while others are lactose intolerant? Why does coffee make me a jittery lunatic, yet some of my friends can fall asleep right after having a cup in the evening? Why do some people get violently ill when they eat wheat, and others consume it with no ill effects?

To answer these questions, we have to go beyond the Blue Zones. Because almost no one alive today has the genes of just one culture, we have to change the way we determine what to eat to live long and be healthy. You don't need to identify your own genome. But you do need to monitor closely how your body reacts to what you eat and what you do. Two decades ago, figuring out what worked was mainly left up to you, and the process could be fraught with assumptions and best guesses. Today, easily accessible science and testing can help you figure out the healthiest way to eat. Finally, a blueprint for your own personal diet is within reach.

To find out how to determine your personal diet, let me introduce you to Chester . . .

# CHAPTER 4

# HOW A HORNY HOG COULD BE THE KEY TO YOUR LONGEVITY

Chester must weigh 500 pounds or more, but he's no taller than my mid-thigh. He's about five feet long with wiry black hair. His ears point sharply forward, nearly obscuring his vision. I've never seen a pig like this.

Rebecca, co-owner of Green Goose Farm and my personal tour guide, says he's a Large Black—a rare heritage breed of hog with an old and well-defined lineage. When he first comes up to us, I'm a little nervous. She's already told me that he sometimes escapes to chase after the females, and looking at the size of him and the flimsy electric fence, I can see how he does it. The fence would be no match for the libido of a Chihuahua, never mind a quarter-ton hog.

But in a moment, he calms my fear by slowly—painfully slowly—lowering himself to the ground and flopping on his side.

"He wants his tummy rubbed," says Rebecca. "Go ahead."

"Me?"

"Yep."

I reach down and rub around his rib cage where it meets his soft underbelly. He grunts with approval. But as enamored as I am of this big lump of cuddle, I realize I'm rubbing bacon in its purest form.

The farm where Chester lives is in Petaluma, California, about an hour's drive north of San Francisco. The ten acres of land used to be an old chicken farm. The remnants of the coops have long since fallen into various stages of collapse, but the farm is thriving, thanks to Rebecca and Roy, her husband and partner. There are animals everywhere: pigs, turkeys, chickens, and sheep—all free to roam about as they please.

I'm here not as an ex-vegan to slaughter a pig or milk some goats. I'm here on a hunch. A few years ago, over a nice dinner at his house in Sarasota, James Williams started telling me about the selective breeding of animals. The topic has been on my mind ever since. Whether you're breeding horses, dogs, or pigs, you can feed them certain foods to make them fatter, skinnier, longer, taller, shorter, or stronger. After a few generations, their babies start to show these traits. The animal's genetic expression becomes part of its lineage. Dogs are the most classic example of this. Your Pug or French Bulldog didn't exist before selective dog breeding for certain traits became popular in the late 1800s. Most dog breeds are only 150 to 175 years old, according to James. It's amazing how fast their genes can change, he says.

After our conversation, I started thinking about how we humans eat and how our genes express themselves so we become fatter, skinnier, taller, shorter, or stronger. After a few generations, we, too, can change our gene expression or even our genes, just as dog breeds have. What this means is that as we change genetically as individuals, our diets may need to change as well.

The work of Weston Price may be the best observational study of this to date. In the 1930s, inspired by his belief that dental health was an indicator of overall health, the noted dentist traveled the world to compare the dental health of Westerners to that of indigenous people.[1] He found that the indigenous he observed had better tooth structure and palettes than the more "evolved" Europeans and North Americans. Not only that, Price noted that many of these so-called primitive people were less likely to suffer the diseases that were ravaging the modern world at the time, such as tuberculosis and diabetes. He attributed their better health to a diet of whole, unprocessed foods. The takeaway is that our advancements in food preparation and preservation are very likely doing us more harm than good, adversely affecting our gene expression.

But even in the face of this evidence, we humans aren't around long enough to actually see the results of changes in our genes. We live long and reproduce late. So while we can observe 2 to 4 generations of our kind, farmers who raise animals like sheep, goats, and pigs can see 10 to 15 generations in as little as a decade. This is gene-morphing gold.

I'm here at Green Goose to find out what Roy and Rebecca, who raise these animals in a traditional, sustainable way, think about my latest theory. Which is that we're no different than Chester, and we can look into our future—our potential genetic success or failure—by studying the challenges facing Roy and Rebecca in raising their animals. If I can learn how feeding and breeding change or maintain the animals' behavior, physical capabilities, and gene expression, I can extrapolate from that how we humans need to tweak our diets to thrive.

I believe that much of the confusion about diet comes from the fact that so many people adhere to a one-size-fits-all approach. *The paleo diet will work for everyone since it's how our ancestors naturally ate,* or *The raw food diet is the answer because it's how humans ate before they discovered fire.* While some aspects of these diets work for some people, other parts of them won't work at all. Why? Our genes. We've evolved from our chimpanzee and Neanderthal ancestors. According to studies at Harvard Medical School and the University of Washington, we've retained only 2 percent of our Neanderthal genes.[2] Genetically, we're worlds away from our Paleolithic ancestors.

The reason one person can happily eat things that would make another person deathly ill is that their genes are different. So if you know how your genes are expressing, you can transcend the diet fads and theories and find the diet that is uniquely beneficial to you. We can eat virtually any diet—vegetarian, vegan, paleo, raw food, all-bacon—that our genes will allow, and live a long and healthy life.

## The Proof Is in the Impotent Hog

Roy walks up to Rebecca and me with a bucket.

"Have you talked about compost?" he asks. So far my tour with Rebecca has given me the impression that these two take the principles of sustainability, permaculture, and farming to a new level. What Roy has in the bucket merely affirms it.

"In here are rumen contents from the sheep," he tells me. "Partially digested grasses and whatever." Roy collected this rumen from the stomach of a sheep they culled—slaughtered—the day before. He explains that since they're putting in a new septic system on the property, he's going to inoculate it with the rumen, with the help of the lamb that is now on its way to a dinner table somewhere in Sonoma County. "If we weren't putting it into the septic tank, we'd use it to help break down the compost."

Their practices inspire envy in even the greenest of Berkeley liberals. But I'm not here to talk about compost; I want to talk pigs and sheep. I want to know what Rebecca and Roy can share that supports my theory. Do they see animals suffer over a few generations with certain feeds? Can they change the size or shape or behavior of animals just by what they feed them or how they breed them? If so, then surely that's happening to us, too.

Absolutely, Roy says. "What we found is that with a heritage breed that's designed to grow slowly on grass and a high-fiber diet—lots of good vegetables, good fiber, a good source of protein—the animals grow slowly, and they're healthy. They don't have a lot of inner body fat. Whereas if you take a heritage animal or a modern breed and you feed it grain, it actually messes with their breeding cycle. They don't breed. I don't know if you saw the boar: he's long and thin. If we fed him grain and kept him confined he probably would not be viable. He would be too heavy, and he'd actually lose the ability to inseminate a female. In six months he wouldn't be any good. The beauty of working with animals on a farm is that in just a couple of years, you can see which traits are inherited versus which are environmental."

We can't see this as easily in human beings, Roy explains, "because our culture masks a lot of what's actually happening with us physically and mentally." He finishes by buttressing my theory: "The same thing has happened to humans as has happened to farm animals."

Rebecca and Roy then tell me about the dairy sheep they got from a friend. The sheep were bred to want grain instead of grazing as they naturally would. They would whine when they didn't get grain. Roy and Rebecca decided not to breed them, knowing that they would just get more sheep with the same hankering for the farmland equivalent of McDonald's. Then Roy tells me about a sow that sat on two litters, killing all her piglets. She was culled for fear that her babies—if any survived—would be equally bad mothers. On the farm, undesirable traits don't get a chance to move into the next generation.

The amount of anecdotal evidence I've amassed about genes expressing or changing from one generation to the next is enough to convince me that the wrong diet not only can change the way an animal looks and acts but also can literally make its lineage die out. We generally don't sit on our babies, but there's little doubt that diet can affect our fertility.

So how can you keep your lineage on the planet? More specifically, what should you eat next time you sit down for dinner? Determining what gene mutations you have and how they can affect your health is a long, complicated, and confusing process. I'm all about shortcuts. And luckily there is one.

How your body is faring can be found in your blood.

## A Snapshot of Every 12 Months or So in Sarasota, Florida

I'm lying on a medical examining table with my left butt cheek exposed. My medical mentor James Williams is filling a syringe with a mixture of methylcobalamin and 25-hydroxyvitamin D3. These may sound like steroids or growth hormones or other serious stuff to you, but they're really only vitamins. Vitamins B12 and D to be specific.

He looks over his glasses at me. "Ready?"

I nod.

He inserts the needle into my glute. It's not painful but also not pleasant. It's 2012, and I'm in James's office for my annual checkup.

Every year he orders two dozen or so blood tests. My local lab performs the tests, then sends James the results to review. After that, I fly down to Florida to see him.

We've just finished going over my results and have agreed that an injection of B12 and D would bring up my low-ish levels. This is the third or fourth year in a row that I've done this with James, and his protocol has saved my health, perhaps even my life.

It was James who discovered how deficient in nutrients and hormones I was after the vegan and raw food diet, along with other dietary shortcomings, by using the blood-testing protocol he's refined over 30 years of practice and more than 100,000 patient visits.

These are not the blood tests you get with an ordinary physical. Those are based on an antiquated understanding of how to use blood testing. While James performs the standard complete blood count, the tests he uses are designed to look at your health long before things go wrong.

## Why Don't All Doctors Use These Tests?

From the time the first blood testing laboratory opened in 1896, in a tiny room at Johns Hopkins Hospital, there was a surge of interest in clinical pathology to diagnose disease. But it wasn't until the 1970s and 1980s that functional medicine specialists like Sheldon Hendler and Jeffrey Bland turned blood testing into a way to determine the future health of a patient. For me, my blood test results represented tangible, unbiased data affirming that my diet wasn't working for me. After seeing my first results in 2009, James urged me to eat more animal foods, something I hadn't done in six or so years. I resisted at first but eventually decided that not having energy, having my body cramp up all the time, and always being on edge was too much suffering. I caved.

Since I didn't want to eat meat, I broke my vegan diet first with goat's yogurt. It tasted amazing. So amazing that at one point I was eating two 32-ounce containers a day. It was excessive but apparently what my body needed, supplying the nutrients I had denied it for so long. After a few months of this, my interest in yogurt waned, and I went on to the harder stuff: meat. I thought the first time I ate meat again would be traumatic and might make me physically ill. But that first taste of chicken in the chicken soup Annmarie's sister made ranks in the top-ten most enjoyable bites of food in my life. I was defeated as a vegan, but I was healthier for it, as my follow-up tests showed.

At the end of my veganism in 2009, my cholesterol was 111, which is very low. By April 2010 it had jumped to 146, and by 2012 it was 175—a little higher than I'd like, but my good cholesterol (HDL) was 75 and the bad (LDL) was 91. The ratio between the two, 1.2, was excellent—a better marker for heart health than total cholesterol.

Another example of how my health improved when I quit the vegan diet is the dramatic increase in my pregnenolone level. When we first tested my level in 2009, it was at 5, equivalent to the level of an 85-year-old man. (I had the libido of one as well.) Clearly I was having some serious adrenal issues caused by my diet and stress. By 2012, after my diet change, my pregnenolone was up to 111.

Over those first few years of testing, it was relieving to see the results go from low to great, since I loved eating just about anything as long as it was organic. But then in January 2014, my test results brought me back to earth. I had gone too far.

My cholesterol had clearly taken a turn toward the negative when the test showed a total of 222. Even worse, my good cholesterol had dropped to 55, the bad had surged to 156, and the ratio was 2.8—still in the acceptable range but a dramatic increase nonetheless. My pregnenolone had fallen to 77, and other levels were askew. My anything-goes, farm-to-table diet was failing me. Blood tests don't lie. I was unhealthy again.

## Ending the Diet Wars for Eternal Internal Dietary Peace

In 2011, I hosted an online event called the Great Health Debate. (You can listen to it at www.GreatHealthDebate.com.) The idea was to gather some of the world's most prominent vegans, vegetarians, and meat eaters to debate the merits of their particular diets. Good idea, but it was nearly a disaster. The event almost never got off the ground because of all the behind-the-scenes bickering. Some experts didn't even want to be in the same state as one another, let alone together on a phone call. So I had to modify the plan. I decided that on the opening night, I'd have a discussion between two doctors who had already agreed to be together—Joseph Mercola, an osteopath who specializes in nutrition, and holistic physician Gabriel Cousens, founder of the Tree of Life Rejuvenation Center in Patagonia, Arizona. I planned to record the other participants separately and play the audios one after another for a week.

Ultimately, the purpose of the program was to show that most healthy diets are pretty much the same and that most experts agree 80 to 90 percent of the time. Second, I wanted to demonstrate that based on gene expression, the remaining diets aren't always the same. And finally, I wanted to challenge listeners to get their blood tested and see if their diet was really working for them. You literally can test any diet you want and see if it's right for you long term. Blood testing stops the dietary debate before it starts.

So here's what's involved:

- **Find a functional medicine practitioner.** You can ask around in your community or go to www.FunctionalMedicine.org for a local listing.

- **Get your blood tested.** If your doctor doesn't have a lab on the premises, you will need to use a third-party lab.

- **Review the results with your doctor** and agree on dietary changes you need to make.

- Commit to making the changes you agreed to.

- **Repeat this process once a year,** or if you're monitoring a health challenge, every three to six months.

Your practitioner will give you a list of blood tests to be performed, or you can take James Williams's list of recommendations to the lab. (See **Recommended Blood Tests and What They Measure.**) Our Complete Blood Test Blueprint Program teaches you how to read your own blood tests. (Go to www.RenegadeHealth.com/bloodtestblueprint.)

## RECOMMENDED BLOOD TESTS
## AND WHAT THEY MEASURE

Physician James Williams, my medical mentor, recommends that you have the following blood tests, which measure important markers for disease and indicators of systemic functioning. A complete workup like this can help you spot trouble before it starts, as well as determine what diet is right for you:

**Complete Blood Count with Differential and Platelets (CBC):** Provides an overview of your blood, including indicators for immune function and markers for anemia.

**Chemistry/Metabolic Panel:** Looks at basic metabolism markers like essential mineral levels, blood sugar, and kidney and liver function.

**Lipid Panel with LDL/HDL ratio:** Checks cholesterol, including HDL (good), LDL (bad), and **Thyroid Stimulating Hormone (TSH):** Checks for under- or overactive thyroid. If the TSH is out of whack, a doctor will suggest further thyroid tests.

**Cortisol, AM Fasting:** Indicates how your body is dealing with stress.

**DHEAs:** Tests levels of hormone that has wide-ranging benefits, including boosting immune system, slowing aging, improving mental function, easing menopause symptoms, and increasing energy, strength, and muscle mass.

**Pregnenolone:** Indicator of adrenal function and overall hormone production, which are often compromised by stress.

**Hemoglobin A1c:** Marker for diabetes.

**Insulin:** Another marker for diabetes.

**Homocysteine:** Heart health marker.

**C-Reactive Protein (Cardiac):** Another heart health marker and general marker for inflammation, a known cause of disease.

**Vitamin B12, serum:** Important vitamin for neurological health.

**Vitamin D, 25-hydroxy:** Important vitamin for bone health, immunity, calcium absorption, and more.

**Iron:** Essential mineral that carries oxygen in blood to organs. Too little (anemia) causes physical and mental fatigue. Too much increases risk of liver disease, heart disease, and organ damage.

Bear in mind that one round of testing will show you only where you are at the moment, not where you're going or where you've been. You have to repeat the tests at least once a year to spot any trends indicating that levels are improving or worsening. If I had stopped testing in 2012, I would have thought I still had great cholesterol, pregnenolone, and DHEA markers, but my 2014 tests showed that this wasn't the case. Seeing the results over time was convincing evidence that much of what I was eating had to go.

It takes more than just eating like someone from the Blue Zones to optimize your diet. Your blood tests will help you unveil what you need to eat that is specifically right for you. Using the data gathered by your yearly tests to make dietary and supplemental adjustments is your clearest path to longevity.

## One More Thing to Consider

There is one lingering issue about what to eat that your genes can't fix. Our world has changed dramatically over the centuries, and our air, water, and food are no longer pristine. While you can see the smog hovering over Los Angeles, you can't see toxic metals like lead and mercury or chemicals like benzene and 1,4-dioxane in your home, your groceries, and your supplements. It's gotten to the point where chemicals like flame retardant are commonly found in baby food, peanut butter, and other staples on the supermarket shelves. This scares the crap out of me. And it should do the same for you.

You could be eating what you think is the best food on the planet, but your blood tests could show signs of disease and imbalance, and you would have no idea why. This is why in a moment of all-is-toxic neurosis, I decide to send everything we were feeding our almost two-year-old son, Hudson, to a lab to test for heavy metals.

The results are surprising, as you'll see next.

# MY CONTAMINATED KITCHEN CABINET: A SURPRISING RESULT

I'm at my desk reading a certificate of analysis for 13 foods we eat at home. I had sent these foods off to a lab a few weeks before to have them analyzed for heavy-metal toxicity. As I flip through the pages of the report, I'm relieved to see that most of the levels seem to be relatively normal—until I get to the sixth item.

What I see surprises me. Lead: 1,570 ppb (parts per billion).

I look at that number again to make sure I read the measurements correctly. This level is higher than the lead in any of the other samples.

*That can't be right,* I think. I check the top of the page to confirm which food it applies to: green tea, one of the best-known superfoods on the planet, one that medical experts and health gurus alike agree is healthy, hype-free, and good for daily use. In fact, I've drunk green tea every day for the last two years. The particular brand we had tested is one that I've used for at least seven months. Could it really have this much lead in it? Or, to back up a bit, is this much lead even a big deal?

It's been a geeky dream of mine to test all the foods my family and I eat for the presence of toxic chemicals and metals. You can't see them or, for the most part, taste them, so it would be a shame to think that we're eating healthy at home and then find out that all the healthy food was actually contaminated.

But now I'm faced with the reality that something I never imagined would be contaminated might, in fact, be exactly that. I expected the rice I sent to have arsenic in it—that has been all over the news. And I thought the seaweeds might have high levels of mercury. But green tea? What else in my cabinet contains levels of heavy metals unsafe for my family and me?

## The Potential Dirty (Almost) Dozen

I'm walking through the grocery store, looking at my list of foods that Annmarie, Hudson, our cats, and I eat regularly. I've decided, for the sake of cost, to send only ten items, nine of which I'll find here. The remaining item will be sushi from the takeout place a block away. I've decided to test only for heavy metals instead of for other toxins like pesticides and endocrine disruptors. Doctors, health experts, and the media almost unanimously cite heavy metals as harmful.

The test we've chosen identifies levels of four of the most toxic metals found in food: mercury, cadmium, lead, and aluminum. It's more than a bit unnerving just how dangerous these metals can be and how easily they get into the body.

- **Mercury** is probably the most familiar heavy-metal toxin, because of widespread warnings about its presence in seafood and dental fillings. Mercury attacks the kidneys and the nervous system, and is a known cancer agent.

- **Cadmium** is used in the manufacturing of all sorts of electronic products, especially batteries. OSHA, the Occupational Safety and Health Administration, estimates that in the United States, 300,000 workers in fields like construction, welding, and recycling are regularly exposed to cadmium.[1] That's not good at all, as cadmium can cause cancer and seriously impair cardiovascular, neurological, and reproductive functioning.

- **Lead,** found in the earth's crust, has a long history of use. Ancient Romans used it in plumbing, and it remains a big threat to our health because of its ubiquity. Lead leaches into the drinking water in houses with lead pipes. Lead-based paint is found in homes painted before 1978 and in furniture painted before 1976. Many toys and decorative objects imported from countries with fewer restrictions contain lead. Like mercury poisoning, lead poisoning is cumulative. Even low levels of exposure over time can cause kidney damage, neurological problems, and developmental disorders.

- **Aluminum,** like lead, is found in the earth's crust. What you may not realize is that foil wrap and pots and pans are not the only sources of aluminum exposure. Numerous foods and medications, including flour and aspirin, contain aluminum in ostensibly safe amounts. But ingest or inhale too much aluminum, and you could find yourself with brain or bone disease.

My hope is that nothing I send to the lab contains high levels of any of these metals, but as I walk through the aisles grabbing items and crossing them off my list, I wonder what I'll do if something does, particularly if it's something that Hudson eats. I'm pretty sure I'll be angry at a whole bunch of people, including farmers, industrial leaders, politicians, marketers, and whoever else has contributed to allowing toxins in our food.

I unload my basket at the checkout counter and check off the items:

- **An organic baby smoothie pack.** This brand, in this flavor, is one of Hudson's favorites. He drinks one or two a day.

- **A packaged seaweed snack from Korea.** Both Hudson and Annmarie eat this. They go through one to four packs a week.

- **Cashews.** Another of Hudson's favorites. He eats them once or twice a week.

- **Organic oats.** Hudson eats these for breakfast three to five times a week.

- **Dulse.** Another seaweed, this one from the East Coast of the United States. Hudson snacks on this once a week.

- **Goji berries, a popular superfood from China.** Hudson eats these two to four times a week.

- **A bag of dried cat food.** Might as well see if our cat, Jonny 5, and B, my brother's cat who lives with us, are safe. Animal food is a huge, underreported problem, causing illness that could be avoided. The cats eat this brand every day.

- **A name-brand baby rice cereal.** I've seen many news reports about arsenic in rice and wanted to see if this mainstream company managed to come in clean. We don't feed this or any rice cereal to Hudson, but I included it to broaden my inquiry beyond foods that health-food lovers consume.

- **A name-brand baby formula.** We didn't feed this to Hudson either. But it's made by a non-organic company I secretly want to catch peddling heavy metal–laced, processed food.

After I pay, I walk to the sushi place. Along with my usual rolls for lunch, I order an extra roll so I can send a sample of the rice off to the lab. I don't eat many deep-water fish, so I'm not concerned about my exposure to mercury in tuna, but I'm worried about the arsenic levels in the rice. We eat at the sushi place often enough that a bad test result would convince us to get our California rolls somewhere else.

At home, I put everything in a box, then realize I can't send it yet, as I don't have the lab submission sheet. I contact Lisa, our assistant, who assures me that the lab will send the sheet to us soon. This delay turns out to be fortuitous in terms of my own heavy-metal exposure.

## 212 Chemicals

Reviewing some research I've done in the past, I come across an alarming report—a 2005 study by the Environmental Working Group[2] that found 287 chemicals in the umbilical-cord blood of ten randomly chosen infants. We're talking about everything from pesticides to waste from coal-burning plants, a nasty group of chemicals, most of which are toxic, cause cancer, or give rise to birth defects.

This means that our second child, due in a few months, will start life with a long list of toxic chemicals in his or her tissues. Mind you, in trace amounts these chemicals aren't necessarily harmful. But I'm bothered that they're there in the first place.

How does a baby get exposed in utero? Unfortunately, exposure comes from mom. Toxic substances she's exposed to go straight to the womb through the umbilical cord. We encounter these chemicals every day. They're in our glasses and plates, and the walls of the buildings in which we live, work, and shop. They're in the air, as well as in our water and food. A 2009 bio-monitoring survey performed by the Centers for Disease Control and Prevention[3] came back with results that mirrored those of the baby study: traces of 212 chemicals were found in the 2,500 study participants, including some particularly dangerous ones like flame retardants, the aforementioned cadmium, and perchlorate, a chemical used in making rocket fuel!

We're all contaminated, but how do we pick up all these toxic substances? If you're indoors, you need look no further than the room you're in. Hormone disruptors are found in plastics[4] and cosmetics. (Cosmetics are tested only for the safety of the finished product, not for the raw ingredients that go into it.) Pesticides find their way into your home from the produce you buy at the supermarket. Heavy metals are in everything from baby formula to deodorant.

There are dozens of categories of substances that are toxic to the body, some affecting us more than others. Heavy metals are high on the list, and among the biggest "carriers" of these are deep-water fish. In 2008, when *The New York Times*[5] analyzed bluefin tuna being sold in some of New York's highest-rated sushi restaurants, it found levels of mercury high enough for the fish to be legally removed from the restaurants. This came a year after a 2007 survey by the New York health department[6] found that one in four New Yorkers had elevated blood mercury levels, closely associated with eating fish. These elevated levels could be especially problematic for pregnant mothers, potentially causing cognitive delays in their children. But increasingly, people who've shifted to a diet heavy in fish, thinking it's healthier, are falling ill from mercury poisoning.

Pesticides and insecticides used in farming practices are also well-documented sources of environmental toxins, linked to a host of disorders. In a paper entitled "Exposure to Environmental Toxins and Agents,"[7] published in October 2013, the American Congress of Obstetricians and Gynecologists warned that such chemicals are potentially harmful at every stage of reproduction. Prenatal exposure increases the risk of childhood cancer; in adult males, exposure is linked to sterility and prostate cancer; and for women, pesticides can interfere with every aspect of reproductive function.

Numerous studies show that nasty toxic chemicals interfere with how our hormones operate.[8] Unfortunately, exposure to toxins like BPA (bisphenol A) is constant, since they're present in most plastic bottles and food-storage containers, and even in the lining of cans.[9] BPA has been linked to erectile dysfunction, heart disease, type 2 diabetes, depression, memory loss, breast cancer, and asthma.[10]

But the word about BPA is out, so you'll see plenty of plastic bottles and containers sporting fancy BPA-free labels. Unfortunately, one of the popular replacements is bisphenol S, or BPS—a derivative of BPA that can be just as toxic to your hormonal system. A study published in 2011 in the journal *Environmental Health Perspectives*[11] found that more than 450 BPA-free plastic products sold in stores like Walmart and even Whole Foods leech estrogenic chemicals, especially when exposed to heat.

## TOXIC CHEMICALS:
## WHO'S WATCHING OUT FOR OUR HEALTH?

So why, you might ask, doesn't someone do more to police the toxic chemicals that turn up in the products we use every day? Technically, the U.S. government does. In 1976, President Gerald Ford passed the Toxic Substances Control Act (TSCA) to regulate new and existing chemicals that might be harmful to "human health and the environment"[12]—particularly those that might cause cancer, birth defects, or genetic damage. The law authorized the Environmental Protection Agency (EPA) to oversee compliance.

In theory, TSCA provides comprehensive safeguards. But in reality, the EPA has tested only 200 of the approximately 84,000 chemicals now in the TSCA registry. (And those 84,000 chemicals are only a fraction of the millions of chemicals currently in use.) Critics of the current legislation—including me—say it protects the companies that make the chemicals, not the people who are unknowingly exposed to them.

When Ken Cook, president of the Environmental Working Group (EWG), an independent watchdog group, gives his "10 Americans" speech—about the 200-plus toxic chemicals the EWG found in the umbilical cords of ten fetuses—he points out some of the glaring flaws in the toxic substances legislation:[13]

> The law hasn't been amended once in the past 30 years, even though tens of thousands of new chemicals have been introduced in products we use every day.

> When the TSCA was passed, it grandfathered in 62,000 chemicals without any testing to prove they're safe.

> Chemicals used in the United States still aren't required to undergo health and safety testing before being put on the market.

> Since 1976, only five chemicals have been banned or restricted under the TSCA.

In May 2013, Congress introduced a bill "to reauthorize and modernize"[14] the TSCA, acknowledging that Americans had lost confidence in the government's ability to regulate chemical use. The main thrust of the bill is a revision of TSCA's subsection S. 1009, the Chemical Safety Improvement Act, that would give the EPA more muscle to test chemicals before they enter the marketplace, rather than following the "safe until proven dangerous" policy that is presently in place.

As it stands, TSCA is "a law that protects polluters," Ken Cook states in a YouTube video of his "10 Americans" speech. "It's a law that protects companies. It's a law that protects profits."[15]

What this means is that to protect ourselves, you and I are the ones who need to police what comes into our homes. There's no one who can do that better.

### Three More, Just for Fun

Again, I'm at a grocery store with a list.

This time, I'm in Calistoga, California, for our Annmarie Skin Care team retreat. It's two weeks after I packed up the box with the food to be tested, and I still haven't sent it. I'm on my way to the post office, but while I'm at the store, I wonder if there's anything else I can add. I remember a friend suggesting that I send the goat's milk and yogurt we feed Hudson, so I grab a container of each. Additionally, I grab a box of my favorite Chinese green tea—the one I'm about to find out contains much higher levels of lead than I'd ever imagined. I add the new items to the lab worksheet and overnight the box to the lab.

### Are You Sure You Did This Right?

After getting back the results of the heavy-metal test a few weeks later, I ask Lisa to schedule a call to the lab project manager, Lydia, who ran the tests on my organic green tea, the last-minute addition that turned up the most interesting results. I want to see if the result is correct beyond any doubt. I have Lisa contact a few food-toxicity experts as well, since I know that any lab technician is going to shy away from questions about whether a food with a certain amount of contamination is toxic. It's a liability for lab technicians to make any statements like that.

On the phone two days later, Lydia confirms that most of the foods I sent have undetectable levels of heavy metals or levels too low to get an accurate reading. This simply means that there's not enough to worry about. This is good news for those foods. We can still eat them.

Then we review the results for the green tea, rice, and seaweeds: the lab report shows higher numbers in these foods for one or two of the metals. The seaweeds and rice each have higher arsenic. And one of the seaweed products has high cadmium, too. As for the green tea, Lisa confirms that they tested it three times. Apparently, when they saw the test results, they were sufficiently surprised to rerun the test to verify the findings.

Lydia mentions that as a regular green tea drinker, she, too, is curious about this number. I let her know that I'm going to purchase three more organic green teas and send them for testing, to see if my brand was just an outlier, or if green tea has an affinity for lead. If the particular organic tea from China I've been drinking contains more lead than other green teas, I'm going to switch, and switch fast. After the call, I buy organic brands from Hawaii, Brazil, and Japan and have them shipped to the lab.

## But Wait: Are There Actually Metals in Me?

A few days later, on my walk to work, a thought pops into my head: *What if I have lead poisoning?* Since there's a relatively high level of lead in my green tea, it would be smart to see if my body is harboring any. To find out, I order a hair-testing kit for Annmarie, Hudson, and me. Hair sampling is said to be a kind of early-warning system, showing disorders before they appear in the rest of the body. This type of test measures the amount of heavy metals in hair follicles. Hair tests are at the front line of heavy-metal testing, though they're still not accepted by the medical mainstream.

We get the kits, cut our hair, put the cuttings in the envelope, and mail them back to the lab. These tests are not meant to measure how much heavy metal is in the body. That's an impossible feat to do while you're alive, because someone would need to analyze all your tissues. The test simply compares your results to those of others who've taken the test. The premise is that if your hair contains high metal content, you have metals in your body as well.

A week later we get the results. What's not great news is that Annmarie and Hudson are both in the 95th percentile for cadmium, which is high. (Hudson also shows high levels of arsenic.) I call James Williams to ask what this means and what we should do next. He tells me that a hair test is just a start. We'll need another test to confirm the results. In James's practice, if the hair test shows positive, he'll follow up with a blood or urine test, or both. If two out of three are positive for heavy metals, that's enough evidence for him to move forward with a metal-detox protocol. I mention the levels of cadmium in the seaweed snacks, but he's quick to tell me that while it may be relevant, the cadmium may be from something entirely different.

The good news is that none of us has a high level of lead or mercury. This means I haven't suffered any ill effects from the lead in my tea. To compare my results, I find the hair heavy-metal test I took in 2010. Almost all the levels are lower now—a positive sign.

Based on the hair test, I'm not thrilled about Annmarie and Hudson's results. But for myself, I've confirmed that the lead in my green tea hasn't ramped up my lead levels. I'll be interested to see if any of the other brands I sent off to the lab contain less lead.

### The Final Results

I had told myself that if one of the other green teas I tested contained less lead than my brand, I would switch. Since the body accumulates heavy metals, why not choose foods that have less? That's just a common-sense approach to reducing the toxic load in your body.

The other approach is to detoxify your body from existing contamination. Unfortunately, detoxing from metals isn't as simple as drinking a little more water than usual, or taking a pill. It's a step-by-step process. Fortunately, physician Mark Hyman, a leading functional medicine expert, has an effective three-step detox plan he uses with his patients. Check out the full protocol at www.drhyman.com.

Further research on the lead in my green tea suggests that many Chinese food products, including herbs, have levels like the one I found, or higher. I asked Carl Winter, director of the FoodSafe program at the University of California, Davis, if I should be concerned about food from China. He declined to single out China, merely saying that certain parts of the world—particularly less developed nations—"are laden with environmental contaminants and these can get into the foods." So it seems I should think about where my food originates, avoiding food imported from countries where farming and manufacturing are not well regulated.

The other green teas I had tested show that there is a lot of variation in the amount of lead in green teas. The one from Brazil had 96.2 parts per billion; from Hawaii, 1,790 parts per billion; from Japan, 69.7 parts per billion. I decide to switch to the Japanese brand, thereby dropping my exposure to lead in green tea by 2,252 percent. When I ask James what level of exposure to heavy metals he considers allowable, he shoots back, "For my patients, the level is zero. Any time you can get purer product, this is better for your health and better for your future health."

Overall, the food toxins experiment was a success. Based on my findings, Annmarie and I decide that each year we'll randomly pick a few things we eat regularly and send them off for testing. In the meantime, besides switching out my green tea, we also eliminate the seaweed snacks for Hudson and ourselves, because of the cadmium. The other seaweed, dulse, tested lower in metals, and it will do just fine. As for the cat food, the amount of lead was elevated. Not enough to warrant alarm or mandatory recall but high enough—based on my green tea results—to start searching for a brand lower in metals. My fear is that we'll have to test a bunch of foods before we find the one best suited to the cats.

## HOW TO REDUCE EXPOSURE TO TOXINS

The best way to reduce the toxin load in your body is to take in as few as possible in the first place. Here are some prevention tips:

**Buy a water filter.** Many chemicals, including chlorine and fluoride, are in our water systems. To avoid ill effects, install water filters on your taps, particularly the kitchen faucet and shower.

**Limit the use of plastic in your home.** You probably can't completely escape BPA and its derivatives. But wherever you can, replace plastics with glass or ceramic containers, dishes, and bottles.

**Use natural cleaning products.** Stop spreading toxins on your walls, windows, and floors. Look for nontoxic cleaning products at the health food store or order them online.

**Open your windows.** The Consumer Product Safety Commission warns that the air inside our homes and offices may be more polluted than the air outside. Keep your windows open when you can. Letting in a little fresh air could save your life.

**Change your beauty products.** Check out the ingredients in your beauty products on the Environmental Working Group's Skin Deep website (www.ewg.org/skindeep/) or read Annmarie's blog: www.annmariegianni.com.

**Eliminate pesticides.** A simple Google search for "homemade natural pesticides for gardens" will reveal a world of nontoxic solutions.

**Eat organic.** This is still one of the best ways to lower your intake of pesticides and heavy metals like cadmium.

## Changing Isn't That Bad

Ultimately, my amateur consumer investigation revealed that toxic chemicals and heavy metals really do appear in our foods. They're not from a tale made up by health nuts or wacky naturopaths. They're not just in someone else's town or country. They're in our hometowns—even in our homes. Right in our cabinets, next to our walnuts and quinoa. Right in our refrigerators—in our fish, eggs, and meat. Which is where this exploration takes me next.

Back in January 2014, when I set out to reexamine everything I'd learned about health and find out what truly promotes longevity, I told myself I was going to do everything I could to get back in shape by doing what gave me the largest returns with the least amount of effort. As of March 2014, the plan was working. I'd lost more than 15 pounds.

Even so, I never thought my journey would take me where I went next—to one of the most uncomfortable places any ex-vegan could be.

# CHAPTER 6

# THE CURIOUS THING ABOUT EATING ANIMALS (AN EX-VEGAN PERSPECTIVE)

Over the countertop, Monica hands me a name tag, an apron, and a towel. With a big smile, she tells me the class will start in five minutes, and I can wait on the bench by the entrance. I look over to where she's pointing and see a few men in their mid-40s sitting with their aprons on, tied in the back. I put mine on and head to the far end of the bench. I'm not in a talking mood.

"Oh, you forgot your cup," Monica says, as I'm about to sit down.

I walk back to the counter, and she hands me a large clear plastic cup, probably 16 to 20 ounces. I'm stumped. I don't know what it's for, and as an ex-vegan taking my first—and possibly last—class in butchery, I'm a little nervous.

"What do I need a cup for? Is there really that much blood?" I ask.

My stomach turns a bit. Maybe it's for just that—in case I get queasy. Or maybe it's where I put all the undesirable parts: sinew, glands, ligaments. I start to think this is a really bad idea.

She laughs and points to a faucet. "It's for water in case you get thirsty. Go grab some before we start."

I like Monica, who I later find out is the co-owner of the butcher shop. But without realizing it, she's put me on edge. I skip the water and sit down. It smells like meat in here. Gamey.

During the almost six years I was a vegan, I was never militantly against other people eating animals, but I did make it clear that their steak came from what had once been a living, sentient being with eyes and a brain that ate, slept, and played with its friends on the farm. (At least that's how it should have been.) At presentations around the country, I would proclaim that anyone who wanted to eat animals responsibly should become intimate with the process of turning them into meat—should get as close as possible at least once. Watch the animal as it's culled or gutted or butchered. My hunch was that if they did this, they'd likely eat less meat—maybe none at all—which would be a victory for me and my vegan cause.

But that was a few years ago. Since then, the situation has changed dramatically.

So this is why I'm here at the Local Butcher Shop—yes, it's actually called that—a few blocks from our house in Berkeley, California, taking a lamb butchery class. I'm reluctant in many ways, but I'm also doing the best I can to stay true to my own word and getting intimate with the process of how animals turn into the meat on my dinner plate. And while I'm not actually killing—sorry, the industry term is *culling*—the animal, I'm getting closer than ever before.

Since I've been eating meat again for a couple of years, the ethics of it isn't a new struggle. But the fact that something needs to die for me to eat it still makes me uneasy. The fact that I may be one of the few ex-vegans who absolutely loves eating meat doesn't make it any easier. I love the taste of it. I love grilling it. I love pig parts and oven-roasted chicken. I love sweetbreads. So, I'm torn.

When it comes to eating meat and other animal foods like fish, eggs, and milk, I want to find out: Do we need these for protein? And if so, is saturated fat really bad for you? Does eating animal foods raise your cholesterol to unhealthy levels? What do all the supermarket labels on meat mean anyway? Is organic the best, or is there better? And, finally, if I have to eat animals or animal products for my health, what are the best kinds to eat and how much should I eat?

Monica asks us all to gather around the butcher table behind the counter. Aaron, her husband and co-owner of the shop, explains that we're going to turn a lamb carcass into lamb chops and other cuts we can take home with us. After he says this, everyone applauds except me. Then, as if on cue, his two assistants, Corey and Bill, bring the headless body from the back of the shop and maneuver it so it rests on the table, its stiff hind legs pointed directly at me.

## Now It's Getting Serious . . .

A lamb is a baby, but this doesn't mean it's small. The carcass is five or six feet long, and it weighs just under 50 pounds. It's a mix of marbled reds, pinks, whites, and yellows—blood, muscle, sinews, ligaments, and bone. As I look at it, I can't help thinking that this lamb died 6 months into its life, and compare that to the fact that Hudson is 18 months old.

Bill reaches underneath the table and pulls out a U-shaped hand saw, the kind I used on metal pipe when I worked at a hardware store and did handyman jobs on the side. I cringe. There's a dead lamb on the table, and I'm going to cut into it and help turn it into chops, leg of lamb, lamb roast, lamb sirloin, and various cuts I'm sure I never knew existed. I'm way too much of a wimp for this.

## An Argument for the Vegan Diet from an Ex-Vegan

Six years of meat-free eating led me here. I started eating vegan after reading about the health benefits. Unlike many other vegans, I wasn't motivated by an animal rights agenda. I started to feel for the animals later. What convinced me that the vegan diet was the pinnacle of all eating philosophies were the hundreds of stories I heard of remarkable healing.

I've spoken to some of the people who got better. Their stories are real. And if you don't believe me, you can read thousands more testimonials and studies on healing with a vegan diet from holistic physicians like Alan Goldhamer and Gabriel Cousens; wellness activist, cancer survivor, and author Kris Carr; and nutritionist Vesanto Melina and dietician Brenda Davis, authors of *Becoming Vegan*. To me, all this was evidence that eating as close to the bottom of the food chain as possible is good for our health.

Take John McDougall, a physician who had a stroke at age 18 that left him endlessly curious about what really makes us sick. McDougall set up a practice in the Hawaiian Islands, where he witnessed first-hand how younger islanders who strayed from the plant-based diets of their elders ended up sicker and more obese. These observations led him to begin treating disease through a low-fat vegan diet, with the result that thousands of his patients were able to reverse their diabetes, high blood pressure, obesity, and more.

The healing power of eating plants is well documented, which makes arguing for eating animals more difficult. But it's not an either/or affair. Putting your health ahead of the life of another animal requires serious consideration.

But if vegan is the pinnacle of all diets, why is there such buzz about nutrient deficiency in long-term vegans? Susan Schenck, author of *The Live Food Factor,* one of the most popular books to spring out of the raw vegan movement, was in the same situation I was. Despite her enthusiasm for the diet and numerous speaking engagements tied to her book's success, Susan slowly came to believe that veganism was undermining her health. She began to experience bloating, deficiencies in vitamins B12 and D, and memory loss. It got so bad she even forgot her husband's cell phone number. At that point, she realized she needed meat in her life. It wasn't long before she was writing another book about her experiences, appropriately titled *Beyond Broccoli.*

Are people like Susan and me doing the vegan diet wrong? Or is the diet itself a poor long-term fit for our DNA?

## Eating Animals: Everyone's Doing It

Bill is cutting through the midsection of the lamb with the saw. It makes a hollow sound as the noise reverberates in the animal's organ cavity. This is all starting to seem medical, like an anatomy class lab but without the smell of formaldehyde. Bill explains that you cut the animal into three sections: the shoulder (the front), the middle, and the legs (the back). He also mentions that they usually use the electric band saw to do this part, so the hand saw is a little old-school.

Once he has the lamb in sections, he puts his hands on the shoulder and legs and looks at all of us. Interestingly enough, there's a shift in how I feel about all this. Because this carcass is no longer a recognizable animal shape, my mind seems to be more comfortable around it. The emotional tension is broken.

I'm convinced that the dissociation I'm experiencing is one of the reasons why Americans have such a meat obsession. According to the United Nations, the average American eats 270 pounds of meat a year.[1] That's a lot. In fact, the only country whose residents consume more meat per capita is Luxembourg. Since meat tastes good and is protein dense, it makes sense that we'd want to eat more of it, at the expense of eating fewer plants. A pan-seared marbled rib eye arguably tastes better than a piece of raw, unsalted, undressed kale.

It's also important to note that there's never been a fully vegan culture. We've eaten meat as long as we've existed. This isn't promising information for PETA supporters. It suggests that somewhere between vegan and our gluttonous American meat obsession, foods from animals are actually a dietary *essential.* According to a paper published by the journal *Nature* in 2013,[2] "The first major evolutionary change in the human diet was the incorporation of meat and marrow from large animals, which occurred at least 2.6 million years ago." Cited as evidence are "butchery" marks on fossil bones, showing where early humans used tools to pry meat from the animals they captured. So, meat's place in our evolution, biology, and overall human experience puts it right up there with sex, water, and air.

Chris Kresser, author of the bestseller *Your Personal Paleo Code,* says there's "quite a bit of research now to suggest that eating meat may have made us human in the first place.

"Before we started eating meat, we had to eat a lot of plant matter throughout the day in order to fuel our energy needs. Meat, however, is a very concentrated, nutrient-dense food source that enabled us to get more nutrients into our bodies faster. This allowed our brains to grow bigger and freed up time for us to do things other than chew plants all day, which is what most primates do. They eat for eight or nine hours a day to support their body weight and their energy needs because they are not eating nutrient-dense foods."

How much meat we need to eat, though, is more difficult to identify. Meat eating in indigenous cultures varies widely, depending on factors like climate and availability. Among hunter-gatherers, the Inuit in northern Canada have a diet consisting of more than 90 percent animal foods, while for the !Kung in southern Africa, meat is less than 10 percent of their diet. Based on the varying rate of meat consumption among our early ancestors, it seems as if we're adapted to survive with varying amounts of meat on our plates. But looking to the early human diet as a guide to how much meat we should eat is as foolish as shaping our own spears to hunt down a deer for tomorrow's dinner. We're not those ancient people anymore. The only thing I've speared in my life is a cheese cube at a cocktail party.

Our modern animal-eating ways began sometime between 8,000 and 6,000 BCE, when hunter-gatherers gave way to early agriculturalists, and goats became the first animals to be farmed.[3] The problem is that our obsession with meat took control of us. It made us take a wrong turn when we decided to remove animals from their natural environment and place them in smaller and smaller areas of confinement. Then we went wildly astray when we decided to feed them foods they would never have touched in nature, in order to fatten them up. When even that wasn't enough, we pumped them full of growth hormones, only to turn around and give them antibiotics when they got sick from the unnatural food and extra hormones. Such is our modern industrial meat system: ugly, cruel, and unhealthy for the animals, as well as for us.

Our little lamb here on the table is one that was easy to catch, but she's an outlier in the animal-eating ecosystem of today. She grew up on a farm no more than 50 or so miles from the butcher shop. She was able to graze freely in a pasture, since her caretakers practice some version of permaculture and organic farming. Unfortunately, animals raised like this are much harder to find than the chicken, pigs, cattle, goats, sheep, or even fish raised on factory farms. The meat from these commercial farms is what we generally eat. The meat from our little lamb on the butcher block and others like it is vastly different from that of a lamb that spent its entire life in a cage, huddled in the same space where it pooped and fed food it would never eat naturally until it got so fat it could barely stand.

## Meat Does Not Equal Meat Anymore

At Green Goose Farm, I asked Roy if his animals ever get sick. Sickness is a sign of an environment and animal in crisis. He said that they rarely do. He explained that their health is directly related to the food they eat—grass, not the grains fed to lambs on commercial farms—and to pasture rotation, which frees the animals from having to forage in their own feces. (To get an idea of the conditions under which supermarket meat is raised, imagine if you were forced to eat Twinkies out of your own toilet.)

Commercially raised animals are sick all the time. According to the Organic Consumers Association, a nonprofit, 80 percent of U.S. pigs have pneumonia when they're slaughtered.[4] In one of my favorite books, *The Omnivore's Dilemma,* Michael Pollan reports that upon slaughter, up to 30 percent of American cattle have abscessed livers, evidence of an infection in the animal's blood.[5]

It is the meat we eat from the hormone- and disease-riddled commercially farmed animals that is making us sick, not the meat from animals that live and eat as nature intended.

For an example of this, we don't need to look any further than the omega-3 content of factory-farmed meat versus naturally raised meat. Omega-3s are essential fatty acids that support cell health, building cell membranes and keeping internal inflammation in check. Our bodies don't manufacture omega-3s: we can get them only from the food we eat. They're found in seafood, nuts, and meat. However, not all meats have the same amount of these essential nutrients. Researchers at the Northern Ireland Centre for Food and Health at the University of Ulster[6] found that omega-3 levels were higher in study participants who ate grass-fed meat than in those who ate meat from animals raised commercially on "concentrate" feed, a mixture of fats, oils, grains, roughage, and by-products of food processing. A 2010 review by agriculture specialists at California State University, Chico, and the University of California Cooperative Extension Service at Davis[7] found that feeding certain breeds of cow a diet of grass instead of grain increases the level of omega-3s in their meat two to five times over.

Think about it: that's two to five times more health-promoting, anti-inflammatory nutrition. So the demonization of eating animals by vegetarians is justified in part: meat from *most* animals consumed by Americans is bad. But a grass-fed, grass-finished rib roast or lamb shank confers health benefits its commercial counterpart cannot provide.

And what about pigs, chickens, and fish? Across the board, every animal raised in captivity has its own nutrient-deficiency issues. Farmed chickens often suffer from caged layer fatigue, a condition in which stress from cramped housing and reduced calcium intake weaken their legs, making it hard for them to stand or walk.[8] Wild pigs root around in the soil with their snouts to get iron and trace minerals from the earth, but they're unable to do that in confinement, so pig farmers have to give them mineral supplements. Sometimes, that's not enough.

## WHAT'S IN YOUR MEAT THAT YOU DON'T NEED OR WANT?

When you buy a rib eye steak from your butcher or supermarket, there's no list of ingredients slapped on the side like you might find on a box of cereal or a can of soup. You'd like to believe what you're getting is just meat, but in a lot of cases it's not. Unless it's grass-fed, grass-finished, and organic, most of the beef, chicken, and pork sold in the United States is pumped full of things to fatten up the animals and keep them disease-free.

**Hormones.** Farmers want their animals to earn as much as possible, so it shouldn't surprise you that most animals bred for meat in America are given growth hormone to make them bigger, or, in the case of cows, to make them produce more milk. The U.S. Food and Drug Administration and the World Health Organization say there's no harm in these hormones, but if that's the case, then why is their safety still hotly debated among medical experts and consumers?

The hormones you're ingesting with your meat and dairy products include steroids—estrogen, testosterone, and progesterone—and recombinant bovine growth hormone (rBGH) to increase milk production in cows. What nobody seems to be addressing is the cumulative effect of these added hormones. According to Craig Minowa, an environmental scientist with the Organic Consumers Association, most of the research is industry funded and finds no risk. However, there are independent studies suggesting a link to certain cancers, he adds.

**Antibiotics.** Farmers regularly administer antibiotics to their food animals to combat the diseases they pick up in the unsanitary and unhealthy conditions on factory farms. In fact, 80 percent of antibiotic use in the U.S. is by the farm industry.[9] This doesn't sit well with people like me who are reluctant to use antibiotics even on themselves. Furthermore, the presence of antibiotic-resistant bacteria is an ongoing threat. A 2001 study published in *The New England Journal of Medicine* found that 84 percent of the salmonella in supermarket ground beef was antibiotic resistant.[10]

It's possible that a rib rack from a lamb raised in a factory farm setting is not even the same food as a roast from a grass-fed lamb. In fact, they may react the exact opposite way in the body, with one causing inflammation—a universal marker for potential disease—while the other fosters an anti-inflammatory response.

## What Is in Meat That We Need?

I'm convinced no one knows for sure what meat contains that we need, but someone who's close is Chris Kresser. I first met Chris at Venus, a small farm-to-table restaurant in Berkeley. He was there with researcher Gary Taubes, author of the bestseller *Why We Get Fat:*

*And What to Do about It.* I didn't know much about Chris then, and he probably knew nothing about me, so after chatting for a minute or two, we went our separate ways.

Two years later, we were reintroduced. By then, Chris's popularity had exploded. His book, *Your Personal Paleo Code*, had made *The New York Times* bestseller list, and his health articles were reaching millions of readers every month. His work combines scientific research, functional medicine, and his experience working with clients at his clinic in Berkeley, where there's a six-month waiting list.

From his book title, it's obvious that Chris is a supporter of the paleo diet, so when I asked him about eating animals, I expected a particular bias. But his personal approach to health and the paleo diet is not a canned, diet-for-the-masses slant, so I knew I'd get some well-researched data. I wanted to challenge him in a way. I know it may be possible to cobble together a diet of supplements, proteins, and plants from all over the world and survive as a vegan, but I wanted him to prove beyond a doubt that this was not a diet for most people if they wanted to thrive.

Chris gave me five reasons why eating animals may help us get healthier: digestible protein, active vitamin A, vitamin B12, iron, and EPA/DHA conversion. Citing a scale called the Protein Digestibility Corrected Amino Acid Score, or PDCAAS, which looks at how many essential amino acids a protein contains, he told me, "Typically, animal proteins are more complete in that respect than plant protein. But this particular index is unique because it doesn't just look at what's in the food; it looks at how well what's in that food is digested and absorbed. Studies using the PDCAAS show that pretty much all forms of animal proteins are more bio-available and more absorbable than plant proteins."

The protein digestibility scale is from 0 to 1.0, with 1.0 being the best source of absorbable protein and the easiest to digest. Chris listed a few protein sources in each category, animal and plant:

**ANIMAL**
Dairy, 1.0
Eggs, 1.0
Light-meat chicken, 1.0
Turkey, 0.97
Fish, 0.96
Beef, 0.92

**PLANT**
Soybeans, 0.91
Chickpeas, 0.78
Black beans, 0.75
Most vegetables, 0.73
Lentils, 0.52
Whole wheat, 0.42
Wheat gluten, 0.25

"It's pretty clear," he said. "If you're looking for digestible protein, animals provide it."

But for all my vegan friends and colleagues whose blood I've set boiling, it's important to note that this in no way means that we need to get *all* our protein from meat. It simply means that animals are a well-digested source of protein. This in some way has contributed to our ability to thrive as a species.

A vegan diet can be challenging for people with certain genetic variations. "There are mutation changes in genes that affect our ability to convert some of the less active forms of certain nutrients found in plant foods into the more active forms of those nutrients," Chris explained. If you can't convert beta-carotene into active vitamin A, for example, you'll end up with a deficiency that makes it difficult for you to see in the dark; drains moisture from your skin, leaving it rough and patchy; and, worst of all, seriously impairs your immune system, making you susceptible to all manner of illnesses and infections.

I was even more convinced of how much we need meat when Chris noted a common problem many of us face: a gut that can't digest plant foods properly and absorb the nutrients we need from them. "Some people have bacteria that make it easier for them to absorb some of the nutrients in plants, whereas other people have a more difficult time extracting the nutrients in plant foods." Often, he explained, the form of a nutrient that's found in plants differs from the form found in animals. Take iron: ferrous iron in plants is harder to absorb than heme iron in meat, putting vegetarians at higher risk for iron deficiency.

People who don't eat animal protein tend to be deficient in B12. Vitamin B12 works with foliate, another B vitamin, in the synthesis of DNA and red blood cells. So a B12 deficiency can cause anything from anemia and fatigue to memory loss, neurological problems, and psychiatric issues. According to Chris, tests have found that 68 percent of vegetarians and 83 percent of vegans are B12 deficient, compared with just 5 percent of omnivores.

Finally, there's the problem that the body can't efficiently convert plant fatty acids into the essential omega-3 fatty acids DHA and EPA. Omega-3s are found in meat, fish, and seaweed but not in plants. They're critical for brain development, they continue to play a major role throughout life, affecting cognition, behavior, and mood. Since the body can't make omega-3s, unless we have an adequate outside source, we'll have suboptimal levels, which, as Chris pointed out, is detrimental to brain health.

Later, when I thought about the evidence Chris presented for why we need to eat at least some animal food, I began to think the reason might not lie in the individual nutrients but in the nutritive value of the whole. There's a little magic on top of the science. Reducing meat to its attributes seems a little like looking at a TV set and proclaiming that it works because of the LED screen or the power cord or the connection to the signal source, totally ignoring the fact that it's all the parts working together in harmony that produces a positive viewing experience.

## But What about Heart Disease or Cancer from Eating Meat?

Back at the butcher shop, we've now broken off into pairs. My partner, Brett, is just as new to this as I am. I contemplate telling him that I'm a recovering vegan but decide I just want to stick to the task. No small talk. I'm deep into the process now. I'm trying to channel my inner hunter-gatherer. It's actually working.

Butcher Corey explains how to separate the femur from the leg muscles. I take the knife and cut along the film that separates the muscle. The muscle easily pulls away from the bone. Once it's separated, Corey instructs me to cut the leg meat into steaks about one and a half inches thick.

Once the steaks are sliced, I lay them out on the butcher block. Shiny, dark red with hints of purple and off-white fat around the edges, the steaks look nothing like the carcass they came from. They look surprisingly familiar and edible. Something you'd see in the supermarket.

They look good to Corey as well. "Nice work," he says. "You can take those home with you, if you want."

Brett agrees that since I sliced them, I should have them.

I nod. I'll take them home, but I'm entirely aware that my new-found skill may have blinded me to the fact that doctors, the media, and vegan-diet experts alike are still adamant that eating meat—red meat, at least—is a direct path to an early grave.

Apparently, the belief that red meat is bad for you can be traced largely to the work of Ancel Keys, an American physiologist who launched the Seven Countries Study, longitudinal research begun in the late 1950s that was the first major study to look at the relationship between diet, lifestyle, and cardiovascular disease.[11] The findings linked coronary disease to a diet full of saturated fat, which is found in meat. In the decades since the landmark study, it has come to be seen as flawed: Keys looked at data only from countries whose results supported his belief. Flawed as the findings were, however, they have stuck.

Chris easily dismantled the assumption that eating meat—particularly red meat with all its saturated fat and cholesterol—is unhealthy. Recent studies "show no association between saturated fat from meat and cardiovascular disease," he told me. "In fact, in many studies, there's even an inverse association between saturated fat intake and stroke, which means that the people who ate more saturated fat lowered their chance of suffering a stroke."

The second myth Chris shot down is that eating red meat causes colon cancer. In a review of 35 studies correlating the two, researchers found no clear evidence of a causal link. Instead, the results indicated quite the opposite: the risk of colorectal cancer from eating meat was actually below 50 percent.

There is, however, a strong link between charred meat and cancer. Meat cooked at high temperatures produces compounds shown to be cancerous. But those same compounds are also produced when vegetables are charred. Chris recommends marinating any food for more than an hour before grilling it, to reduce potential toxic by-products.

### All the Parts

The science behind eating meat seems solid, but I still need to know which animals and which cuts are best to eat, and how much we should be eating. Standing in front of a growing pile of fat, discarded bones, sweetbread, and cartilage, I can see why tribal people ate the whole animal. It would be wasteful to discard these calories if I was a true hunter-gatherer.

Aaron chimes in to explain that at the Local Butcher Shop, none of the animal goes to waste. They use the fat to make lard and the bones to make nutritious stock. Scrap pieces are ground up for sausage, and the heart, liver, intestines, and any other edible parts are sold. What they're doing harks back to the sacred tradition of honoring the animal for its ultimate sacrifice by making use of it all.

As queasy as I still am about getting closer to the killing and gutting, I support the practice of wasting none of the animal's precious contribution. Whether you're spiritual or not, using the whole animal makes eating meat more practical in terms of calories, nutrition, and dollars saved. If you eat only muscle meat, you don't get the same nutrition as if you include organ meats and bone broth in your diet, according to Catherine Shanahan, medical consultant to the L.A. Lakers and author of *Deep Nutrition,* who has studied traditional eating habits in many cultures. But if the idea of eating organs turns you off, a quick glance at the menus of some of the world's fanciest restaurants might change your mind. Blood sausage, liver, bone marrow, and sweetbreads are very trendy right now—and chock-full of nutrients. Heart is low calorie and low fat, and it's full of amino acids and compounds that support the production of collagen and elastin, which help your skin stay supple and youthful. Heart can be cooked in stews, or sliced and sautéed with mushrooms and onions. Bone broth is used as a base for soups and stews and is a traditional healing remedy. It contains gelatin, which helps digestion, and glycosaminoglycans, which aid joint health. It's also said to boost immunity. Liver and kidneys are nutritional powerhouses, full of protein, iron, CoQ10, and vitamins A and B12. Kidneys are also low in fat.

## WHAT DO THOSE LABELS ON MEAT MEAN?

If you decide to include meat in your diet, make sure it's from high-quality, naturally fed animals. This is not always easy to guarantee. It can be frustrating trying to decode the labels in the meat section of the supermarket:

**U.S. Department of Agriculture (USDA) Certified Organic** indicates that the animal was not treated with antibiotics or hormones and had some outdoor access, though it may not have been much.

**Cage-Free** means the animal was not confined to a cage, but still it was very likely raised on a factory farm under stressful conditions. The Cage-Free designation is not regulated by the USDA.

**Free Range** means meat and poultry were given outdoor access, though it may have been for no more than five minutes a day.

**Pasture-Raised** means the animals were raised outdoors and allowed to graze or live some semblance of a natural life. If you see this designation, it's worth checking out the farm online to see if the animals really are being pastured.

**Grass-Fed** indicates that cattle were raised on a natural diet of grass, not grain feed. But some farms grass-feed their animals initially, then move them to a pen and finish them on grain. So make sure the label says grass-finished, which means the animal was able to forage its entire life up until slaughter. And look for the label USDA Process Vertified, to make sure the farm's practices are up to your new level of diligence.

### Eating Animals: Fewer Is Better

I've concluded that animal protein is an essential part of the human diet—or at least of my diet—but I still don't know how much to eat. Here again, the longest-living modern cultures might provide a clue.

What's common to all the Blue Zone cultures, notes author Dan Buettner, is how little meat they eat compared to people in North America and most of Europe. Most of them reserve meat for special occasions, which for the Sardinians includes Sundays. The people of Ikaria, Greece, serve goat on special occasions but eat a lot of fish. Okinawans eat both meat—usually pork—and fish, but sparingly. The Seventh-Day Adventists in California are largely vegetarian; the few who eat meat serve it only as a side dish. The Nicoyans in Costa Rica are the only Blue Zone culture to eat meat regularly, but even they consume far less than the average American.

So, regardless of what diet you choose, eating more plants and fewer animal products seems to be the takeaway from the modern longevity studies. I still believe some food from animals, possibly even beef, lamb, or pork, is a necessity for most humans, but if you feel you're destined to eat only plants, give it a shot. There are ways to work the vegan diet so that you get almost all the nutrients your body needs. I said *almost:* you may still find you're deficient. I strongly advise vegans to stay away from those gimmicky packaged foods like soy chicken nuggets, steak made from corn protein, and mock turkey made of wheat protein and soy. These products are notorious for their poor digestibility, genetically modified protein, additives, and low nutrient value. Eat real food.

I also urge you to remember that a diet of only plants has its place as a healing diet because what you leave out—processed foods, genetically engineered soy, hormone-laced dairy—is more significant than what you leave in. This is why the vegan diet or even a raw food diet can be so healing as a short- to medium-term therapy—from a week to a few years.

But whatever diet you choose, I want it to work for you. The only way to know if your diet is working is to assess your results by running regular blood tests and working with a practitioner who knows how to read them. For vegans, low iron, low hormones, and too-low cholesterol are among the first places to look for a clue that your diet is taking you away from the health and longevity that you're after. Monitoring your health is equally important if you're eating animals. If your nutrient and hormone levels are low, you may need more meat in your diet. But if your levels are on the high side, you may have let your meat obsession take control of your diet.

## FISH: FRIEND OR FOE?

All this talk about little lambs and enormous and friendly hogs is very interesting, but what about fish? Where does your piece of grilled salmon fit into the debate about eating animals?

The truth is, fish are nutritional powerhouses: high-protein, low-fat sources of essential nutrients—omega-3 fatty acids, vitamin D, and selenium—that promote heart health and cognitive function. And the good news is, you don't have to load up on fish to get big results. Just one or two servings a week will lower the risk of death from heart disease by 36 percent, researchers at the Harvard School of Public Health found.[12] Other studies show that the same amount of fish can also protect against stroke and depression, boost immunity, and reduce inflammation.

EPA, an omega-3 in fatty fish like salmon, halibut, cod, and sardines, lowers blood pressure and cholesterol. DHA, another omega-3, supports brain development in babies[13] and, at the other end of life, protects the aging brain against Alzheimer's disease and dementia.[14] Researchers found that seniors who ate fish one to four times a week actually had more gray matter than non–fish eaters in brain areas related to memory and attention, and in the orbital frontal cortex, which is involved in critical functions like "social adjustment, and the control of mood, drive, and responsibility, traits that are crucial in defining the 'personality' of the individual."[15]

But do the benefits of eating fish outweigh the risks? There's concern about contaminants like pesticide residues, preservatives, and polychlorinated biphenyls (PCBs) turning up in your fillet of sole. In 2003, the Environmental Working Group found that 70 percent of farmed salmon were tainted with PCBs, dioxin-like carcinogens.[16] But after industry cleanup efforts, salmon are now considered safe to eat. Mercury poisoning remains the greatest risk to fish eaters: it can lead to nerve damage in adults and stunted brain development in fetuses and infants.[17] Unfortunately, guidelines on how much is too much mercury are all over the map. The best advice is not to order sushi every night and to avoid seafood that carries a greater risk of mercury contamination, like swordfish, shellfish, white meat tuna, and warmwater fish. Essentially, you want to stay away from the big fish that eat a lot of smaller fish, since mercury accumulates in their tissues. Wild-caught salmon, halibut, cod, sardines, and anchovies are safer.

I recommend avoiding farmed fish like the plague. Fish farms are like factory farms but underwater. The fish are crammed into cages, pumped full of antibiotics and dyes, and fed on grain, which no self-respecting salmon would eat in the wild. "Organic" farmed fish don't fare much better. So, go wild, go smaller, and enjoy your fish dinner.

## One Last Lesson from My Lamb

It's closing time at the butcher shop. I pay up for the class, and they hand me 18 pounds of lamb meat that will last up to six months or so in the freezer. On the way out the door, I replay something Rebecca and Roy said: that the only reason the heritage hogs on their farm have survived as an old-world breed is because they're bred for meat. Otherwise, their lineage would have been eliminated because of the commercial demand for pigs that are genetically programmed to fatten up fast and yield more meat per dollar.

About a block away from home, physical reality knocks me out of my meat-eater's nostalgia. This bag is getting heavy. I'm glad I don't have to drag the whole lamb home to my family, as my hunter-gather ancestors would have done. With that, I start to ruminate on what type of exercise we're supposed to be doing.

I've always assumed walking and running are the most natural ways to exercise. But just as we've lost the knowledge of what foods we're supposed to eat, are we equally confused about what exercise is best for us?

I get home to find Annmarie and Hudson already asleep. I check my email and find an ominous message from a friend who months earlier, in the name of fitness, convinced me to participate in a Tough Mudder adventure race with him and four other friends. There are only a few weeks to go, and I'm beginning to think that even though I want to reach the pinnacle of personal fitness, Tough Mudder is not the way to go about it. The photos in the email attest to that. They show event participants struggling to get through a dozen or so obstacles, ranging from jumping into ice-cold water to running through dangling live electrical wires—which is exactly where you'll find me next.

# CHAPTER 7

# EXERCISE: ALMOST EVERYONE DOES IT WRONG; HERE'S HOW TO DO IT RIGHT

The first electric shock isn't so bad—it feels like a hard pinch, but the surface of my skin is hot.

*I can handle this,* I think.

But I can't. When the second shock hits, my vision goes black. For a split second, I can't hear the crowd around me. Everything slows down, like I've entered a time warp. Then, just as quickly as everything dialed down, it speeds up again. My vision clears. My hearing comes back. My feet must have left the ground when I was zapped, because now they land in a puddle with a splash, as I stumble through the rest of the dangling electric wires. One more shock hits me, and then I'm on the other side.

It's late May 2014, and I've just completed Electroshock Therapy, the last of the obstacles on the ten-mile Tough Mudder course. This event has exploded in popularity among extreme athletes, reinvented couch potatoes, and everyone in between.

I'm here in Vermont with my childhood friends, to kick-start getting back in shape. We gather quickly at the end of the race to look back at what we've survived. *Being shocked repeatedly in the name of fitness can't be healthy,* I think, and believe me, this isn't the first time I've felt this way today.

## Rewind One Hour and Eight Minutes to the Arctic Enema

It's a little over an hour earlier. At an obstacle called the Arctic Enema, I'm jumping into a tank of 36-degree water. This water isn't just cold. It's frigid *and* dirty: light brown like a creek after a heavy downpour. The objective is to jump in, fully submerge yourself, duck under a wooden beam in the middle of the tank, then come up on the other side, climb out, and continue on the course.

As an ex-personal trainer, I'm a little confused. This isn't fitness; it's torture. I take a deep breath and plunge into the icy water. This confirms beyond a doubt that many of us will do really weird things in the name of fitness.

The Tough Mudder has a much higher risk of injury than a run around the neighborhood. An emergency room team studying participants in a Tough Mudder race found the number and severity of injuries "unusually high," with racers risking "permanent disability."[1] I'm doing the race anyway. I've been brainwashed into believing that fitness has to be ridiculously hard and painful to be worthwhile. This misperception started back in high school and persisted long after I hung up my football cleats and left organized team sports behind. If it didn't hurt, you weren't trying hard enough. Though the "no pain, no gain" mantra has probably produced more injuries than champions, I still think I need to push beyond my own physical limits to see results. To prove it, I'm submerged up to my neck in miserably cold water.

The reason I'm here is that after Hudson was born, I decided to eat in excess for a bit and desperately wanted to lose that weight. Essentially, my weight gain made me extremely susceptible to influence, and I was talked into this. But the truth is you don't need to climb a 20-foot wall with the help of a knotted rope, crawl on your belly under barbed wire, or endure electric shocks to enjoy the benefits of exercise and fitness. The secret to exercising right is not to work *more* but to work *less.*

## Have Legs, Will Run

I'm convinced there is a species-specific exercise that all humans are physically and genetically built to master. And the natural fitness activity for us humans doesn't include fancy machines or swimming in the Arctic Ocean in late January. It's gimmick-less, simple locomotion—walking, running, and jumping. But as simple as running is, if we understand our biology as runners and the physiology of running, we can apply that knowledge to make the most of just about any exercise we want to do.

If you don't believe that we were meant to walk or run, you have to look at the obvious logic here. What was your ratio of kettlebell swings (or bench press reps or box jumps or crunches) to footsteps today? I'm sure the footsteps exceeded the kettlebell swings by a multiple of thousands. Even if you pushed back the clock 10,000 years, it would be a similar ratio, minus the kettlebells. We were made to walk and run. Our survival depended on it.

Studying the history of the human predatory nature, biologist Bernd Heinrich, author of *Why We Run*, looked at traditional cultures in Africa and determined that our ability to hunt prey depended on our slow-twitch endurance muscles, which allowed us to outlast the animals with fast-twitch, sprinting muscles that we were trying to kill for food. We hunted by stalking our prey until they couldn't run any more. Endurance also puts us at a psychological advantage, Heinrich says.

"We are psychologically evolved to pursue long-range goals," he writes, "because through millions of years that is what we on average *had* to do in order to eat. To us, even an old deer that had not yet been caught would have required a very long chase." People who were unsuccessful at this hunting strategy "left fewer descendants,"[2] he explains.

What happened to the deer or rabbit we caught is the same thing that happens to marathon runners who go out too fast and hit "the wall," barely able to move another step. Their muscle glycogen stores are depleted by the exertion, and they build up more lactic acid in their bodies than they can burn for energy. Something similar happened to the Neanderthals, Christopher McDougall writes in *Born to*

*Run.* Bigger and stronger than our fleet-footed running ancestors, the Neanderthals were at a disadvantage, especially in hotter weather, and were easily outrun by their prey.[3]

Together, McDougall and Heinrich come up with a convincing set of biological arguments, including muscle makeup and lung capacity, for why we humans are born to run. But if this is the case, we've gone pretty far off track. If running is so natural, why do so many people get hurt doing it?

## America's Great Exercise Confusion

After I read Heinrich's book ten years ago, I took his advice to heart. On a suggestion from a friend, I signed up for the Hartford Marathon, never having run more than ten miles in one session. At that point, I was running three or four times a week and bicycling 25 to 50 miles every weekend, so I figured my body would be able to meet the challenge of running 26.2 miles. After all, I reasoned, we are *built* to be runners.

The result was miserable. I finished the race but with a strained calf muscle that required eight months of rehab before I could get back in my running shoes.

This sort of thing happens way too often, because of our all-or-nothing approach to fitness. We either do it or we don't. And when we do it, we do it way too much and hurt ourselves, and when we don't do it, we really don't—in fact, we even lie about it.

A 2008 study by the National Institutes of Health[4] found that despite saying that they exercise, most Americans do not. Less than 5 percent of the 6,000 people surveyed got the recommended amount of exercise—30 minutes, five times a week. Another study, released in 2013 by the Centers for Disease Control and Prevention, found that 80 percent of Americans weren't getting the recommended amount of exercise.[5]

And those who exercise are overdoing it, just like I did. Particularly those who run. "The data suggests up to 79 percent of all runners are injured every year," Stephen Messier, director of the J. B. Snow Biomechanics Laboratory at Wake Forest University, told Christopher

McDougall for an article in *The New York Times*. "What's more, those figures have been consistent since the 1970s."[6]

These stats aren't in any way appealing to someone who wants to get up off the couch and run.

They're not very appealing to those doing other types of exercise either, because the injury rates are high for many other popular forms of exercise. A 2014 study of CrossFit athletes found that about 20 percent had suffered injuries.[7]

Even if you don't injure yourself, you may put way too much stress on your body. Technique is to blame for many injuries, it seems. We may be born to run, but we do it wrong. In his *Times* article, McDougall pointed to common missteps like landing on our heels and failing to push off with our toes. Heavy on our feet, we blame it on our shoes. "We don't need smarter shoes; we need smarter feet," he explained. While training in Mexico with the ultramarathoning Tarahumara Indians, McDougall jettisoned his shoes and adopted their "whisper-soft stride."[8]

In my own first marathon, I made a classic American exercise mistake: I put my mental conditioning before my physical conditioning. I overstepped my body's boundaries at the time, which is a form of overtraining. Overtraining is something my fitness Yoda, Phil Maffetone, built his entire career on—at least until he decided to quit and become a songwriter.

### Musician? Chiropractor? Guru?

A trained chiropractor who never considered himself one, Phil Maffetone was a well-respected holistic doctor with clients like singer/songwriter James Taylor and Mark Allen, a six-time world champion triathlete. But after two decades in Westchester County, New York, Phil decided to close his successful practice and pursue songwriting. Working with celebrities, endurance champions, and people just looking to get healthy wasn't enough to keep him practicing. What did, though, was a phone call.

Five days after he closed his practice, Phil got a call from a man named Rick. Rick had read some of Phil's books and wanted to get on a program. Phil resisted at first, but Rick persisted—at least enough to reveal his last name: Rubin.

Rick Rubin is arguably one of America's most successful music producers of all time, with a client list that runs from Tom Petty, LL Cool J, Beastie Boys, Metallica, and Kanye West to Ed Sheeran, Josh Groban, and Adele. Working with him was an opportunity Phil couldn't pass up. Phil said he would help Rick with his health if Rick would help Phil with his songwriting.

Rick agreed, and Phil moved to Los Angeles. Over time, Phil ended up not only working with Rick but also becoming the personal physician to the Red Hot Chili Peppers and Johnny Cash. Along the way, he learned songwriting and has since produced four albums, with contributions from clients like John Frusciante of the Red Hot Chili Peppers.

*The Maffetone Method*, the book I managed to get my hands on after my first marathon, soon became my new fitness bible. I used it to help me get back on track after my running injury, and I still consult it for reference.

I've never trained with Phil, but Annmarie and I met him and his partner, family physician Coralee Thompson, at their home in the southern Arizona mountains in March 2009. Phil has the long gray ponytail of a hippie but the confident directness of a native New Yorker. Even though much of his fitness work has been with champion endurance athletes, Phil's principles apply to all levels of fitness. His commonsense advice to eat healthy, exercise, and reduce stress is genius, because it targets the American obsession with overexercising in a way that's both scientific and easy to grasp.

What causes the largest percentage of injuries, Phil says, is overtraining, no matter what your level of fitness. As I was outlining this chapter, I called him, and he pointed me to an article he posted on the Natural Running Center website about a triathlete named Angela Naeth who came to him with what he calls *overtraining syndrome*. As he explains:

> The overtrained athlete is often exhausted, broken down, and unable to train or race. But this is a late-stage condition of a spectrum called the overtraining syndrome. Early on, less-obvious indications predominate—and this is when the problem

is relatively easy to eliminate. Properly done, this can quickly restore better performances, eliminate injury and fatigue, and improve the body's fat burning state. Reducing training volume and or intensity is often the place to start.[9]

Essentially, Phil's advice is to exercise less, do it more efficiently, and be patient. This, though, isn't what most people want to hear. Clearly, many of my fellow Mudder participants were not patient in their training. While the Tough Mudder may have motivated them to get into (or back into) shape, it was clearly too tough for a number of the participants. If they had been my personal training clients, I would have advised them to work up to the challenge, walking on a treadmill for three months before moving on to more strenuous activity—definitely not starting out with a ten-mile race up and down a ski mountain. As I found out when I ran my first marathon, the quest for fast gains invariably leads to long-term pain, fatigue, and eventual burnout. Even high-level endurance athletes struggle with Phil's advice to slow down. When Angela Naeth came to Phil, she had a leg injury and other imbalances related to training. Phil suggested that she train less for better results, and it worked. Her performance improved, and she has since maintained her status as one of the top female Ironman athletes in the United States.

Angela's success got me thinking. If less really is better, then why on earth do we work out like crazy in the first place? The answer, I concluded, is that we assume we can accomplish more than what we're physically capable of—at least at the time—so we ignore the subtle and not-so-subtle warnings our body gives us. The number-one reason most people cite for exercising, or for resuming exercising if they've stopped, is to reach some short-term goal: weight loss, more muscle, flatter stomach, a toned butt. And there's often a secondary goal behind that, such as looking good for an upcoming event like a wedding or a school reunion.

We're unreasonably attached to our goals, so we hurt ourselves. It happened to Angela and it happened to me, and it definitely can happen to you too.

What's confusing is that most of the science about what works fitness-wise is geared toward these faster short-term results. Sure, you can reach short-term goals in record time—lose that stubborn last ten pounds or strengthen your pecs—but it will be at the expense of your overall long-term physical well-being.

While I'd like to improve my performance, my ultimate exercise goal is part of my longevity plan. The most convincing science about exercise shows that it's beneficial for brain health, cancer prevention, detoxification, stress relief, and much more. And all these benefits point to a longer, healthier life. "A great deal of the physical effects that we once thought were caused by aging are actually the result of inactivity,"[10] Hirofumi Tanaka, director of the Cardiovascular Aging Research Laboratory at the University of Texas at Austin, said in an interview for exercise columnist Gretchen Reynolds's bestseller, *The First Twenty Minutes: Surprising Science Reveals How We Can Exercise Better, Train Smarter, Live Longer*.

The bottom line is, exercise is good for extending your life.

### (Over)conditioning Neo-Native Style

It's October 2010.

Annmarie and I are in Buffalo, New York, for a month, helping a woman named Lauren get into shape. We're filming a monthlong makeover as a mini-documentary for our YouTube channel.

In an attempt to appease my Neanderthal roots and ignore what I've learned from Phil, I get swept up in the CrossFit hype. CrossFit is a high-powered fitness regimen developed by Greg Glassman that is described on its website as "constantly varied functional movements performed at relatively high intensity." It doesn't advertise that its theories of exercise are based on the fitness routines of ancient peoples, but its concepts of building strength and explosive bursts of movement are certainly more Neanderthal than savanna. The paleo diet, which ostensibly has a caveman connection, is the CrossFitter's most popular system of nourishment.

I instantly like Dave, the gym owner, and we sign up for 30 days on the spot. The next day, we're doing a Workout of the Day, aka WOD. What surprises me is that it's only 12 minutes long and consists of just three exercises: 10 dead lifts, 10 burpees (a four-step exercise that involves squatting, kicking your legs back, jumping back into the squat, then standing), and 5 pull-ups (the bicep curl kind)—repeated for as many rounds as possible. My past fitness training makes me skeptical that this is enough to get a good workout, but I soon find out that it's plenty.

Actually, it's too much.

As the 12 minutes expire, I can barely breathe. My head starts to hurt, and I'm dizzy. For the first time, I understand why my friend Mike used to vomit after he ran a race. I go outside, thinking I might do just that. Luckily, the nausea passes, and we get in the car for a 30-minute ride home after being at the gym for all of 18 minutes, 12 of them for the workout. What doesn't go away is my headache, which lasts for 24 hours. Additionally, I did so many pull-ups that my elbows are nearly locked at a 45-degree angle for three days.

This was another classic overtraining experience—exactly what Phil warns against—but I want to be clear that how I felt wasn't Dave's fault. I should have gone at a slower pace that worked for me. Still, there's something wrong with the CrossFit premise if even one round of dead lifts, burpees, and pull-ups—supposedly good for everyone at every fitness level—produces those results. What would happen to an out-of-shape rank beginner? Even a 12-minute workout could start a newbie down a path of overtraining, resulting in more harm than good. As Phil explains:

> When we have too much stress, the body has to go into a different kind of mode to adapt. So when exercise becomes an excess stress, we produce more cortisol—which is sort of our emergency first-aid kit—and this gets us into trouble. We're beating up the body and not recovering from day to day. We develop various problems in the brain and in the body and we break down more easily. We age quicker.

So it's likely that I aged a little from that workout at the CrossFit gym. However, after a few days, Annmarie and I go back and work at a smarter pace for the remaining 29 days we're in town. Still, I'm concerned for others who get involved with a program that encourages fast, high-intensity training. If you don't know your threshold, which is different for every individual, you could end up hurting yourself doing what you thought was good for you.

So what is the threshold? How can you determine if your exercise is working for or against you?

The answer is the number of times per minute your heart beats while you're exercising, no matter what kind of exercise you do.

## The Better Fuel

The Tough Mudder I participated in was at Mount Snow, a popular Vermont ski resort. When I was a kid, I spent plenty of time riding the chairlift up the mountain and bombing down its sometimes snowy, usually icy trails. For this event, they added a lot of mud to the trails, and there was no chairlift to take you up to the summit. Over the ten-mile course, the terrain rose some 3,500 feet, which meant hills—steep ones—and lots of them.

Having run multiple marathons successfully after that first misstep, I learned that when you're running for distance and not looking to win, it's generally best to walk up the hills to conserve your energy. So at mile seven, I was trudging up a seemingly endless hill, feeling tired but good. I didn't burn myself out early in the race, so I was able to maintain a steady pace, passing people on the sides of the trail who were unable to catch their breath.

I was in better condition than they were, but I've been in their position. When we met Sebastian on our first trip to Peru, in 2010, I was the one who was struggling.

We had just finished a healing ceremony with Sebastian and James, and we were about 2,000 feet below the summit of Pachatusan. With our small group of ten, we were following Sebastian up a steep ridge. Annmarie and I were winded after only a few meters. As I stopped to catch my breath, I could see Sebastian 100 yards above me, steadily climbing. He's 20 years older than me and had neither run four marathons as I had nor spent any time in a gym, but he showed no signs of needing a break.

What was happening in Sebastian's body was physiologically different from what was happening in mine, even though we were on the same mountain together. And my research has shown that this difference is why there is so much confusion about what exercise is best. We can all be doing the same type of exercise but running on different fuel. Depending on each individual's heart rate, lung capacity, and level of conditioning, the exercise will be pro-health for some and pro-stress for the rest.

The body has two major fuel systems: aerobic and anaerobic. The aerobic system uses fatty acids, glycerol, and oxygen for fuel; fatty acids and glycerol are formed when fat tissue is broken down. When your body goes into aerobic mode, it burns fat within a very specific range of heart beats per minute. This is known as your fat-burning zone.

If you exercise at too high a heart rate, you will slip into using your anaerobic fuel system, which burns glucose (blood sugar) to fuel your muscles and creates lactic acid. The longer you exercise in this anaerobic state, your sugar-burning zone, the less likely you'll be able to continue. Once more lactic acid builds up than your body can burn, you won't be able to move well. So this zone has a more defined limit than the fat-burning zone. Remember the deer that's chased until it can't run anymore? That's you when you're in your sugar-burning zone. Operating in this zone not only stresses your body but also creates sugar cravings, because you need to replenish the glucose stores you've depleted.

We seem to be addicted to getting into this anaerobic mode during exercise—pushing the body past its ideal aerobic limit. This is what happened to me at the CrossFit gym. It's not all a foolish pursuit: there is some science saying we burn more fat and calories in the sugar-burning zone. But it's important to note that exercising in the sugar-burning zone is not beneficial for long-term health, causing stress that is more damaging than any short-term benefit gained. Phil reminds me that our long-term health goal is to eliminate stress, not to put ourselves under more stress. This quick-result, short-term approach to fitness is like using our body's fossil fuels. They burn well and generate a lot of energy, but eventually they run out, at the expense of our body—our "planet." In ecological terms, this approach to fitness is unsustainable.

So why not use sustainable forms of energy instead? The aerobic heart-rate range burns fat and creates less stress. Doesn't that seem like a better option?

"You need to train your metabolism to be a better fat burner," Phil says. "Those who burn more fat, relying less on sugar, are not only healthier but become fit more easily."

So fat burning is where it's at—*regardless of the type of exercise you choose.* I want to be totally clear about this. Some of the people climbing the hill at Mount Snow were in the sugar-burning zone, causing stress to their bodies, while I was in the fat-burning zone, benefiting from the activity. Similarly, climbing the mountain in Peru was the same exercise for Sebastian and me, but his heart was beating slower than mine (and definitely not threatening to explode out of his chest). He's built with a larger lung capacity than mine and is conditioned to take in more oxygen to use as fuel. Sebastian's resting heart rate is in the 40-beats-per-minute range, like that of many well-trained endurance athletes. My resting heart rate, though good, is between 55 and 60 beats per minute.

The same could be said for my CrossFit experience. It wasn't that the exercise itself was excessive. My body just wasn't in the right shape to handle that type of exercise in a fat-burning mode.

---

### WHAT'S YOUR RESTING HEART RATE?

Cyclist Miguel Induran, who won the Tour de France five times from 1991 to 1995, is famous for something else as well: a resting heart rate of 28 beats per minute. That's phenomenal, but a resting heart rate in the 35-beats-per-minute range is not unusual in professional athletes.

To find out your resting heart rate, all you need is a digital watch or a timepiece with a second hand, and your own two fingers.

Step 1. Make sure you've been sitting for at least 60 minutes.

**Step 2.** Turn your left wrist so your palm is facing up. Place the index and middle fingers of your right hand on the soft tissue at the right side of your wrist. Feel around until you find the pulse.

**Step 3.** Looking at your watch, count the number of beats in a 15-second period. Then multiply that number by four. That's your resting heart rate in beats per minute.

Most people have a resting heart rate of 50 to 80 beats per minute. If yours is 80 or more, wait 15 minutes and try again. If it's still 80 or above, consult your doctor for a checkup. Elevated blood pressure can be a sign of a more serious medical condition.

The slower your heart beats, the more conditioned you are. Your heart doesn't have to work so hard during exercise, and you're more likely to burn fat, your body's preferred fuel. Less stress on your body can help you realize the important goal of living longer.

The relationship between heart rate and mortality is a subject of fascination to the scientific community. In a now-famous study published in 1997,[11] Herbert J. Levine, a cardiologist at the Tufts University School of Medicine, observed that every species of mammal "from hamster to whale" has a set number of heartbeats per lifetime. The exception? Humans. But Levine's finding led him to speculate about whether by slowing our heart rate we could extend our life expectancy.

One thing that separates modern humans from our early ancestors is our resting heart rate. A lifetime of tracking prey conditioned early humans so that their resting heart rates were much closer to those of elite athletes than to yours or mine. We have been conditioned since birth to spend most of our time sitting, with occasional bursts of activity. The discrepancy between the way we live now and what we were built to do is the source of much confusion among exercise gurus. Endurance advocates say we're naturally meant to run, while high-intensity exercise advocates say we're naturally meant to be doing quick bursts of exercise, not endurance exercises like running.

I think it's possible we are supposed to be doing both high-intensity and endurance exercise, but in order to do them safely, we have to consider the fact that our oxygen intake and heart rate are unlikely to be close to those of our ancestors. So whether you prefer endurance sports or high-intensity exercise, be sure to stay in a heart rate zone that focuses on efficiency, not stress on the body.

### Your Ideal Fat-Burning Heart Rate

There isn't one ideal heart rate we all should maintain. There's a lot of variability, so you will need to find your own optimum exercising heart rate. Generally, a heart rate between 105 and 134 is in the fat-burning zone, according to Gretchen Reynolds. But at this level of intensity, you don't burn too many calories overall, she explains. So if your goal is to burn body fat and calories, it's still best to work out near the top of that zone.

This is fine advice if you're taking a short-term approach, with weight loss or weight maintenance as your main fitness goal. But if you're looking for a longer life, you'll want to train at your maximum aerobic heart rate. To find your ideal training heart rate, based on your age and present state of health and fitness, you can use Phil Maffetone's 180 Formula, available on his website, www.philmaffetone.com/180-formula.

Now that you know that staying within your fat-burning zone is the key to smart, efficient exercise for longevity, you just have to choose a form of exercise.

### So What Are the Rules That Let You Do Any Exercise You Want?

At the finish line of the Tough Mudder, you get two things: a bright orange headband with the Tough Mudder logo on it and a 20-ounce plastic cup of Dos Equis, a Mexican beer. Beer is not the best source of hydration, but after slogging through that ten-mile obstacle course I'd argue it's better than Advil as a short-term painkiller.

I think I'd have felt better if I'd just done an ordinary run. Not necessarily ten miles, but long enough to clear my mind and give me more benefits than just maintaining my weight. Running, for me, is the perfect exercise.

The Q'ero, Sebastian's people, don't run. They hike. And there's no evidence that people from the Blue Zones spend hours in the gym, run marathons, or do anything remotely like an American exercise routine. Their lives are naturally active, so they stay fit. But we're not in the Blue Zones or the mountains of Peru. For most of us, everyday life is sedentary. We can park at the back of the mall parking lot or take the stairs instead of the elevator to our office, but it doesn't replace nine hours of sheepherding. Unless your work involves a lot of manual labor, you'll need to find some sort of aerobic exercise to stay fit. Yoga is a fantastic way to clear your mind and stretch your body, but few forms of hatha yoga—except maybe a vigorous vinyasa—will put your heart rate in the fat-burning zone. You'll still have to do one or two sessions of higher-heart-rate activities a week. Similarly, if you're lifting weights and your heart rate doesn't go up, I'd suggest you add some cardiovascular circuits to your routine. If you do leg presses, for instance, alternate with some box jumps. If you do bench presses, alternate with some push-ups. Lifting weights will give you muscles, but getting your heart pumping will add days to your life. In cases like this, variety in your training will give you the best results.

## Follow the Exercise Rules

Maybe running to you is like public speaking: you'd rather die than do it. Maybe you prefer lifting weights, CrossFit, spinning, tennis, or competitive curling. It doesn't matter what you choose. Almost any form of exercise can be beneficial, as long as you follow certain rules.

**Don't overdo it.** If you want to avoid getting hurt, don't jump into your first high-intensity training class like you're a pro, or do a triathlon on a whim, or run 26.2 miles if you've never gone more than 10. If you're just getting back to exercising, you could start with walking. Most people would be surprised at where their heart rate is after walking briskly up a steep hill.

**Pick a fitness activity you like.** The only exercise you'll stick with for life is one you enjoy. There are fads in fitness as in everything else, so do what you love and keep doing it, no matter what science comes out that discounts it. If an activity involves your feet, legs, and arms, it's suitable for human participation.

**Keep your heart rate in the fat-burning zone.** Don't overdo it, but don't be too wimpy to push yourself once in a while. Be patient: eventually your physical fitness will catch up to where your mind wants you to be. Even endurance athletes take a while to find the perfect training range. "Initially, training at a relatively low heart rate may be stressful for many athletes," Phil Maffetone says. "But after a short time, you will feel better, and your pace will quicken at that same heart rate. You will not be stuck training at that relatively slow pace for too long."

As much as a champion athlete might find it frustrating to train at a slower pace, I imagine you might actually be relieved to take it slow and not work too hard. In the long run, you'll get better results because your body will experience less stress—and when I say stress, I mean the physical kind.

The emotional kind is a little more difficult to manage, but it can be just as damaging to your health. Even with all I know about health, fitness, and stress, emotional stress has given me the most fits as I've attempted to master it. My recurring stress nightmare replays itself every time I travel, as you're about to find out.

# CHAPTER 8

# HOW ONE CRAZY TECHNIQUE AND AN HERB FROM INDIA COULD ADD YEARS TO YOUR LIFE

It's March 2014, and Annmarie, Hudson, and I are in the Denver International Airport. Our flight to San Francisco is delayed four hours. This is a minor inconvenience. We normally book our flights to coincide with Hudson's nap time, so this will just force us to walk him to sleep in his stroller.

After 30 minutes of riding around in the stroller, Hudson is freaking out. He's so tired he can't sleep. Denver International, or any airport for that matter, is not a great place for an attentive, curious one-and-a-half-year-old to sleep. The next three and a half hours are filled with fussing, screaming, kicking, and throwing food.

During this time, I'm a mess—frazzled, pissed off, and snappy. I'm dealing with Hudson's meltdown by having one of my own. In one particularly hectic moment, I look over at Annmarie in total disbelief: she seems just as calm as she would be if she were walking on a beach in the middle of a two-week vacation. Does she not hear Hudson's ear-piercing screams? Or sense his anger and frustration?

"How come you don't freak out when he's acting like this?" I hiss, half-jealous, half-curious.

"I know he's safe, and he's just trying to express himself," she says.

Same situation, completely different perspective, wildly different stress levels. In *The Myth of Stress,* corporate trainer Andrew Bernstein explains that it is our thoughts that stress us out and not the stressors themselves. Just seeing the tiger doesn't cause stress; it's thinking the tiger might eat us. This is exactly what is happening to me at the airport. My thoughts are making me a basket case, while Annmarie's are keeping her calm and stress-free. This is what I now call "The Annmarie Effect."

Finally, we get on the flight, and Hudson falls asleep as expected. Annmarie does, too, while I'm left to slowly process the built-up cortisol—stress hormone—left in my body.

## More Stress at 35,000 Feet

After an unusually bumpy and stressful 15 minutes over the Rockies, I've calmed down enough to think of things other than the plane falling out of the sky. I'm envying the man next to me. The turbulence finally woke him up, but unlike me, he isn't gripping his armrests. In fact, during the worst of the turbulence, he reached into the seatback pocket for the SkyMall catalog. He seems to have not a care in the world. I start to wonder if conditioning has set me up for a slightly more intense fear of flying than I normally have. I'm pretty sure my seatmate was smart enough not to watch a TV show about an Ethiopian Airlines crash in the ocean, as I did about 90 minutes ago. His mind isn't newly wired to be worrying about a dangerous outcome to this flight, as mine is. Unlike me, he's not messing with his longevity by stewing his organs in a cortisol broth.

Cortisol, which is produced in excess by the adrenal glands when you're under stress, is linked directly to inflammation and weight gain—two of the main reasons stress is so dangerous to your health. I'm convinced that you can eat as healthy as you want and exercise perfectly, but if you stress too much you can undo all the good. Stress is perhaps the biggest killer around—even more than French fries and fast food.

It's no secret that people who are stressed out pack on more pounds. From 1995 to 2004, Harvard researchers observed 1,355 men and women to see if there was any relationship between body mass and stress.[1] What they found was a definite association between stress and weight. Men who were under increased work- and home-related stress gained an average of 3.02 pounds, while women experiencing the same stressors gained an average of 3.46 pounds. Those numbers might not seem like a lot, but remember, there were people in the study who gained more than that, increasing their risk of coronary heart disease, high-blood pressure, type 2 diabetes, stroke, and even colon and breast cancer.

Another negative effect of stress is inflammation. Inflammation—a catchall term for an immune response in the body—is partly regulated by cortisol. Research at Carnegie Mellon University[2] found that chronic stress hinders the body's ability to stop inflammation. Sheldon Cohen, lead researcher on the study, had previously found[3] that psychological stress makes us more susceptible to colds. The sniffles seem trivial, though, compared to the real risks of inflammation, which include chronic diseases and conditions ranging from heart disease and rheumatoid arthritis to asthma, colitis, and dementia. Essentially, if there's inflammation, there's probably illness around the corner.

"Inflammation leads to every one of the major chronic diseases of aging," Mark Hyman explains. "It's also by far the major contributor to obesity. Being fat is being inflamed—period!"[4]

Stress, inflammation, weight gain—a triad of health sabotage. And then there's aging. The granddaddy of stress research, Hans Selye, summed up his 50-plus years of study with the observation that every stressful situation leaves its mark, and we pay for it by aging a little faster.

Studies aside, we don't need the experts to tell us that stressing out is bad for us. Just think how drained you feel, physically and emotionally, when you've been trying to juggle pressure at home and at work. Or how anxious you feel when you have to deliver bad news. Or how agitated you are by persistent worry about money. Chronic stress plays an influential role in the long-term decline of your health.

So, given all the evidence I've uncovered about the harm stress can do, I want to eliminate as much stress as possible and face the world—particularly my next plane flight—with the calm of a Zen monk. And I want to use tools that work for me. Finding the stress relief tools that work for you is like finding a life partner. You can try a bunch, but when you find the right one, you know it's a fit. Maybe for you it's meditation or long walks or watching funny movies. Google *stress-relief techniques* and you'll find more than I could possibly cover in this chapter. But since I've had such great results with two that are rather unorthodox, I feel it's only fair to introduce them to you.

This is where a strange technique that involves tapping on my chin and other facial and body areas comes in.

### "What the Hell Are You Watching?"

It's 2004, and I show up at my friend Nick Ortner's apartment in Bethel, Connecticut. We've known each other since second grade, when his family moved to the United States from Argentina.

Nick shows me into the living room, and I sit down on the couch.

"You have to see this," he says, indicating a program paused on the TV. "It's called EFT—Emotional Freedom Technique—or tapping. It was created by this guy named Gary Craig." Nick is pointing to a wiry older man on the screen.

"EFT, phone home," I joke. "I thought we were going to watch the Jets game."

"We will, but this first."

Nick un-pauses the DVD. A man who's deathly afraid of water is standing with Craig about 20 yards from a swimming pool. The goal, Nick explains, is to get this man into the pool using EFT, which I quickly realize may be the silliest-looking technique I've ever seen.

"What the hell are we watching?"

"Just wait."

A few minutes later, my desire to watch New York Jets football starts to wane.

On the screen, Craig has moved the water-phobic man from 20 yards away from the pool to 10 yards away. To get him closer, they've been tapping specific places on their hands, faces, and torsos, while Craig asks the man why getting into the pool scares him so.

I'm skeptical, but it seems to be working. There is noticeable progress. The man is loosening up. Maybe it's not a parlor trick. Nick explains that some people who've been in years of talk therapy see better results in hours, sometimes minutes, with EFT.

Five minutes later, the two men are both on the pool deck. Craig's goal of getting the guy into the water seems almost possible. I'm a little anxious. I want him to get into that pool.

Five more minutes, and Craig asks the man if he'd like to step into the water.

"Whoa," I say out loud.

The once water-fearing man says, "Sure," and dips his foot into the pool. On his face you can see that his mind is blown.

So is mine.

A few minutes later, the man is floating on a pool noodle, playing splash games with Craig. They're giggling like ten-year-olds. I feel like I've witnessed the inner workings of a real-life when-pigs-fly moment. The tapping acted like a pressure-release valve for the man's anxiety. Tap and release. Could it work for stress, too?

## Tapping for Stress

Psychologist Roger Callahan discovered the tapping technique in 1979. At the time, he was working with a patient named Mary, who had come to him for help with a crippling water phobia that had haunted her since childhood. Callahan had tried a variety of techniques, but nothing was working. After a year, Mary was still terrified of water.

The breakthrough for Callahan and Mary came during a session in which Mary told him that simply thinking about water gave her stomach pains. Callahan had been reading up on traditional Chinese medicine and the meridians or energy channels in the body. He knew that the end of the stomach meridian is a point under the eye. He suggested that Mary tap there with her finger. Why not? He had nothing to lose, he figured. Within minutes, Mary was elated, and Callahan was shocked. Her anxiety and stomach pain were gone, and she went outside and sat next to the pool without feeling nervous at all.

Callahan refined his work, eventually calling it Thought Field Therapy, or TFT. Then Gary Craig, one of his students, further refined it and brought it to a larger audience as the Emotional Freedom Technique. Years later, Nick Ortner became a steward of EFT, writing a bestselling book, *The Tapping Solution: A Revolutionary System for Stress-Free Living,* and teaching it to thousands on stages all over the world.

As nutty as it looks, EFT isn't really that far off base. Tapping, which is the commonly accepted name for the technique these days, works because it stimulates acupressure points on the meridians that the Chinese have used in healing for thousands of years, "tapping" into the body's own healing mechanism. It's essentially a non-invasive form of acupuncture, which is very well studied, particularly for relieving stress.

But you don't need to pull out any ancient Chinese scrolls to dig up this research and assume it applies to tapping, too. Dawson Church, a well-known tapping practitioner with possibly the best laugh you've never heard, has already done the work. His team studied veterans suffering from post-traumatic stress disorder to see how an hour-long tapping session would impact their stress levels. Tapping, it turns out, reduced the stress hormone cortisol by an average of 24 percent, with some subjects registering a whopping 50 percent reduction. By comparison, subjects who underwent an hour of traditional talk therapy showed no reduction in cortisol levels.[5]

Somehow the physical act of tapping on meridian points disrupts the brain's signals to the adrenals to churn out cortisol. It may still seem like magic to you, but I assure you it's not.

The science can't show you firsthand how powerful this is, so I asked Nick for some examples of people who had found relief from emotional and/or physical symptoms. He told me about Claire, a mother, grandmother, and loving wife who felt overwhelmed by life. She had tried a number of stress relief techniques, including meditation, yoga, and affirmations, but none had worked. By simply tapping on her feeling of being overwhelmed, she had a mini-revelation—that stress came from her *belief* that nothing ever worked out for her, not the *fact* that nothing ever did, because in truth, things did work for her. She was just focusing on the things that didn't.

Nick also told me about someone we'll call Tina, who had neck and back pain she couldn't seem to shake. She was the caregiver for her 89-year-old father. Nick worked with her for her pain but soon realized that she was also sad and that her father was causing her a lot of stress. Tina was trying to make herself better through new, healthy, spiritual and personal-development activities, but her father judged everything she tried. As the sessions continued, Nick had Tina tap on her father's judgment, and within a few minutes her neck pain was almost completely gone. She experienced relief not only physically but also emotionally. She felt lighter, and realized that the constant stress she associated with her father was gone.

Tapping is pretty amazing, but it isn't the only stress-relief tool I use. The other is one that I forgot to take before I boarded that flight at Denver International Airport. It's just about as close to a magic bullet for finding calm as any I've tried.

## RELIEF FOR COMMON STRESS TRIGGERS

Nick Ortner, author of the bestseller *The Tapping Solution,* has taught thousands of people all over the world how to use tapping to relieve common stressors like the following:

**Trying to be perfect.** The stress that comes with this is never ending. You can never be perfect, so the chase never stops. Tapping on how you beat yourself up for not doing things perfectly is helpful in relieving stressful feelings around perfectionism.

**Family relationships.** Triggers around family are often so deep that they affect our overall stress levels in many ways. Were you told you weren't good enough? Did a parent treat you badly? Were you not given enough attention? Are you the black sheep? Tapping can help release feelings of stress from family tensions and neglect.

> **Setting boundaries.** Few people find it easy to say no. Most of us want to be helpful. Unfortunately, saying yes too often leads to overcommitment, overscheduling, and tension. Tap on getting comfortable with maintaining boundaries and saying no.
>
> **Social media, technology, and the inability to disconnect.** It's almost impossible to disconnect in our hyperconnected world. The solution to dealing with the stress of all this input isn't to turn off your phones, computers, and iThings. We're a technology-driven culture, and that's our future. But spending too much time and energy on media, technology, and social networks is an addiction that takes you away from human connections, your relationships with others. Tapping can help you break the compulsion and become more conscious about your choices.
>
> For a diagram of tapping points and a basic tapping sequence for anxiety, see www.thetappingsolution.com/what-is-eft-tapping.

### "Take This, Maaaannn"

A young man plants himself in front of me. Mid-20s. Brown, unwashed hair with a feather dangling from it. He opens his hand, revealing two brown capsules. I'm convinced this neo-hippy is handing me mescaline.

His hand is a little shaky, and one pill starts to roll off his palm. He stops it with his other hand and looks me in the eyes.

"Here, these are for you. I looove your wooork, bro," he drawls. I realize he's a little nervous, not shaking because he's jonesing for a fix.

"What are they?" I ask.

"They're the best adaptogen on the planet."

"Rhodiola?"

"Naaah, bro, that stuff makes me feel weird."

"Yeah, me too. Ashwagandha? Siberian ginseng?" Now I'm engaged. He's speaking my language. Adaptogens are probably the most interesting of all substances in the health space. They work with the endocrine system to either calm or energize the body, depending on what the individual needs. They can reduce cortisol in your body and, in turn, reduce stress.

"Nope," he tells me. "Holy basil."

"Not sure I know too much about it," I admit. I'd come across holy basil in my research, but there are so many things to learn about that I'd passed it up.

"You will after you take these, maaaaannnn."

So I do. I grab a glass of water, he drops the pills in my hand, and I pop them in my mouth.

"Coooooooool," he says. "Let me know what you think." We shake hands, and he walks off.

I realize how what just happened must look. I took two brown pills handed to me by a stranger at a health conference where half the audience was middle-aged women and the other half 20-something dudes with feathers in their hair.

I hope I can trust this man.

### Two Hours Later . . .

I'm on the rooftop of the hotel. I'm naked. I think I can fly.

Just kidding.

I'm not any of those things. I'm still in the conference hall. But I definitely feel different. I feel as if anything can come my way and I'll be able to handle it in a cool, collected manner.

On my cell phone, I sneak a peek at the entry for holy basil in *Rodale's Illustrated Encyclopedia of Herbs* online. In India, I read, "It is a sacred herb dedicated to the gods Vishnu and Krishna. Sprigs of the species *Ocimum sanctum* (Holy Basil) at one time were laid on the breasts of the dead to protect them from evil in the next world and to offer them entrance to paradise."[6] Maybe I've entered the paradise promised. I thank Vishnu and Krishna. Holy basil is proving very quickly to be the adaptogen for me. These health events are usually nerve-racking, with people constantly coming up to me, wanting to talk and ask questions. Today, however, I'm handling it all like I'm in complete flow.

It's rare to take a supplement and actually feel something. It's even rarer to take one and feel this good. Relaxed. At peace. I have to find this guy and see where he got these pills. I want to share them with our readers on the blog. With my mom, friends. Anyone who'll listen to me.

To date, holy basil is the closest thing to a short-term stress solution that I've found. It is not to be confused with the same basil you put in your pesto sauce, though they are both in the mint family. The plant—*Ocimum tenuiflorum,* aka *Ocimum sanctum* Linn, aka tulsi—has played a spiritual and medicinal role in India, Sri Lanka, and Malaysia for centuries. In *Plants of Life, Plants of Death,* Frederick J. Simoons writes that to the Hindus, tulsi is the most sacred of all plants. Ayurvedic healers regard it with the same reverence Chinese healers reserve for ginseng. Ginseng is a respected headliner on the healing circuit, so if what Simoons says is true, holy basil is like the underground rock star who hasn't yet been discovered.

The Herb Society of America's *New Encyclopedia of Herbs & Their Uses* describes the medicinal properties of holy basil: "a pungently aromatic, warming antiseptic herb that lowers fever, reduces inflammation, relaxes spasms, clears bacterial infections, strengthens the immune and nervous systems. It is considered tonic and adaptogenic, and lowers blood pressure and blood sugar levels."[7]

The range of medicinal uses attests to the herb's reputation for exalted healing powers, ranging from malaria, gonorrhea, and gastric problems to colds, coughs, influenza, bronchitis, pleurisy, asthma, sinusitis, headaches, rheumatism, arthritis, and diabetes. As *The New Encyclopedia of Herbs & Their Uses* tells us, its use extends even to "low libido and negativity." In Ayurvedic medicine, a mixture of holy basil, other herbs, and honey is used to treat "skin and ear infections, mouth ulcers, stings, and bites."[8]

## Trust Me, the Stuff Works for Stress

In terms of stress reduction, what's important to note is holy basil's purported ability to lower blood pressure, reduce inflammation, and treat negativity. It may be a leap to conclude that this herb eliminates stress. But a literature review by Indian researchers confirms the plant's adaptogenic properties, finding "substantial evidence" of tulsi's "significant preventive and curative potential with respect to the stress-related degenerative diseases endemic to industrialized societies."[9]

It's hard not to be excited about findings like that. Unfortunately, the research to date has all been done on animals, as holistic physician Andrew Weil noted in a 2004 blog post. Despite that, he found the evidence that holy basil may counteract the effects of stress compelling. Weil cited an animal study published in India in 1991 that compared holy basil, Siberian ginseng, and Asian ginseng, "and found that holy basil was the most potent anti-stress agent of the three and also had the highest margin of safety."[10]

Based on my personal experience and the experience of thousands of people who've tried holy basil because of our blog, I suggest we don't need to recreate thousands of years of Ayurvedic medicinal history. The herb works for stress. As one person who uses our holy basil extract told us, "It improves my composure, my outlook, my state of mind and overall comfort level, and reduces stress. I feel more balanced and confident just from drinking one cup."

I'm skeptical about most everything, but for me, testimonials like this are evidence that something is happening that you may want to become a part of. Call it a stress-free—or at least less-stress—revolution. It seems to start with holy basil.

## HOLY BASIL: WHERE TO FIND IT, HOW TO TAKE IT

You can find holy basil, also known as tulsi, at most health food stores, or you can order it online. It generally comes in four different forms: loose leaf; dried powder (capsules); leaf extract (capsules or powder); and tincture (liquid). Holy basil is a tonic herb, like ginseng, meaning that it doesn't have ill effects if taken in moderation and it's safe to take over prolonged periods. The standard recommendations for use are:

**For stress relief:**
   **Tincture:** 40 to 60 drops three times a day
   **Loose leaf:** 1 teaspoon in a hot tea as needed
   **Dried powder capsules:** 300 to 2,000 mg a day as needed
   **Leaf extract:** 500 mg a day

**To clear airways in nose and chest and ease breathing:** 500 mg of dried powder (capsules) three times a day

**To help control blood sugar:** 1,000 to 2,500 mg of dried powder (capsules) a day

### SIMPLE HOLY BASIL TEA

1 teaspoon holy basil (loose leaf)
Sweetener of choice (stevia or honey are mine)

Bring water to just under a boil, then remove from heat. Add the holy basil and steep for 3 to 5 minutes. Strain and add sweetener.

## HOLY BASIL CHAI SPICED TEA
## (RIDICULOUSLY GOOD)

**To make the tea:**

1 cup water
1/2 teaspoon holy basil (loose leaf)
1/2 teaspoon fennel seeds
1/2 teaspoon cumin
1/4 teaspoon cloves
1/2 teaspoon cardamom
1/2 teaspoon cinnamon
Pinch of vanilla powder

Combine ingredients in a pot and simmer for at least 20 minutes. Strain.

Before serving, add fresh coconut milk (see below) or organic coconut milk.

Alternatively, if you aren't allergic to dairy, you can add cow's milk and honey.

**To make the coconut milk:**

1 cup coconut water
½ cup fresh coconut meat
2 tablespoons raisins

Blend ingredients and strain through steel mesh strainer.

## The Jab, Then the Upper Cut

You can use either tapping or holy basil for stress relief, but I recommend using them together, to pack a one-two punch. Stress has a way of clouding your thinking, and it's hard to stay calm when a car cuts into your lane without signaling or a family member sets you off. Holy basil, taken daily, helps keep your body in stress-prevention mode. So when stressful situations arise that would normally get your heart pumping adrenaline-filled blood through your arteries, you'll be less reactive. Then, once your stress response is disabled and you're cooler and calmer, you can use tapping for the deeper work of putting out the fire altogether. Holy basil is the jab; tapping is the upper cut, the closing blow.

Of course, just because I find holy basil and tapping invaluable for stress relief, you don't have to use them. Your stress-relief toolbox may be different than mine. Walking, meditation, deep breathing, screaming into a pillow—there are thousands of methods of de-stressing that you can find with a simple Google search. As with exercising, what's important isn't what you do; it's that you find what works best for you and do it.

You won't do it perfectly, whatever method you choose. No one does. So don't stress about it. Or if you do, use tapping to address your stress around not doing your stress-relief techniques perfectly. If you can suspend your inner skeptic for a week, I urge you to try the one-two punch of holy basil and tapping. The worst that can happen is that you prove me wrong. The best? Less stress—and quite possibly a longer life.

Speaking of not doing something perfectly and stressing out about it, next up you'll find me extremely tired of my extreme diet. So tired, in fact, that I'm at the breaking point, wondering if I'm crazy for thinking what I'm doing is right. Or just plain crazy for doing it.

# CHAPTER 9

# SUGAR, CARBS, AND GLUTEN: A HOLY TRINITY OF DISEASE . . . OR NOT?

I'm tired of eating this way.

Every morning for the last year, I've had a bowl of soaked chia seeds, almonds, and stevia for breakfast. For lunch, it's salad with olives and vegetables. For dinner, salad again, usually with sauerkraut, sometimes with tempeh or tofu.

It's mid-2009, we're nearly a year and a half into our RV trip, and I'm at the point of dietary breakdown. I'm no longer a raw foodist, but I'm still vegan. Right now, though, I've gone back to mainly raw food. I'm on a no-sugar, no-carbohydrate diet.

I'm doing this because I'm hopelessly confused about the health symptoms I'm experiencing. I can't get out of bed. I have acne all over my face and back. I'm anxious and moody. I feel like I've tried everything to change, but nothing has worked.

I'm concerned that I have candida, a yeast infection in my gut. From my research, I gather that all these symptoms could be related to it. I took antibiotics for 21 days after finding a tick on my leg and seeing that round, ring-like rash associated with Lyme disease. Around the same time, I was experimenting with a fruitarian diet (yes, only fruit), which could have fed the yeast in my gut, after I disrupted the flora balance with the antibiotics. Finally, one morning after going to the bathroom, I saw what looked like a cotton ball in my stool—a pretty strong indicator of a candida overgrowth, particularly since I haven't eaten cotton balls since I was three. This, of course, freaked me out but also affirmed what I was dealing with. So I embarked on an aggressive anti-candida diet, which essentially meant no sugar, no fruit, and no complex carbohydrates like rice, quinoa, or wheat.

In the beginning it was easy. I felt like I was making progress. My stomach felt better. Some of the acne cleared up. No more yeasty poo balls either.

But after a few months the symptoms stayed pretty much the same. So I pushed on. Now, almost 365 days later, the symptoms are getting worse. I still think it's candida. I wonder if I'll have to do this carb-free diet for life. Forget cake or brownies or cookies, pasta or bread or crackers. I just want a piece of fruit. Not even fruit with a ton of sugar but something low-glycemic like a blueberry or a raspberry.

The way I'm eating now doesn't feel right, but I can't break down now and give up. Eventually, I feel, I'll break through the issues I'm having. This diet will do it. I know it.

## It Didn't Do It. Fast-Forward Four Months

The amount of goat yogurt I'm eating now is insane. Sometimes I eat it plain, sometimes with blueberries, sometimes with bee pollen. Almost always with honey. *When* I eat it doesn't matter to me. I can do yogurt at breakfast, lunch, dinner, or all three. I'm convinced this may be the world's most perfect food.

Annmarie warns me that it could cause some serious health issues if I continue to eat 64 ounces of yogurt a day. I don't care. My body needs it.

I'm off my carb-free diet, and I'm starting to feel better. Looking back, somewhere between Day 1 and Day 365 of that diet, I made a mistake. It's highly likely that there was candida in my gut, but it wasn't there the whole time. I *did* get rid of it with my carb-free diet, but my mistake was that after it was gone, I kept on thinking that my symptoms were from the candida infection, not from something else. When James identified my adrenal and hormonal issues, convinced me to stop being vegan, and put me on some targeted supplements, my symptoms started to go away—fast.

Restrictive diets like the one I just suffered through are terribly challenging to stick to, and it's relieving to know that I don't have to be on a carb-free diet my whole life. Not having fruit or rice or quinoa for an extended period of time is self-imposed torture. If the diet were an interrogation technique, I would have confessed to a crime I didn't do.

So what is it with sugar and carbs, which break down into sugar? It's no secret that people around the world love carbs. Carbs can define entire cultures. Who are the French without their bread, Italians without their pasta, Chinese without their rice? We love sugar, too. Not only is a piece of ripe, sweet watermelon the definition of a summer BBQ, the strawberry shortcake for dessert is just as iconic.

Both sugar and carbs are everywhere, and for many people, they're the most difficult things to keep away from. Studies show they can be as addictive as coffee or cocaine. Ever since the rise of the Atkins diet and, more recently, the paleo diet, sugar and carbs have gotten a bad rap. Based on how some diet gurus demonize sugar and complex carbohydrates, you'd think eating rice would have wiped the Chinese off the planet, but they're still here. So are carbs really as bad for us as some diet experts want us to think?

Many of us, including me, are pretty confused about what to do when a basket of Italian bread and a bowl of fresh olive oil are placed in front of us at our favorite restaurant. Too many carbs? Too much gluten? Should I save my calories for the sugary tiramisu I want for dessert? Or is that forbidden, too?

Truth is, that single combination of bread and oil may be a small representation of the reason doctors, researchers, health experts, and the rest of us are so scared of sugar and carbs.

To find out why, I want to introduce you to Tom.

## A Para-Cyclist with a Rare Genetic Disorder
## Explains Everything

I've never met or spoken to Tom Staniford, but he seems like the type of guy I'd like. Tom was born with a rare genetic disorder called mandibular hypoplasia, or MDP syndrome, which doesn't allow his body to store any fat. Only eight people in the world have it. Because of MDP, Tom's face and body are literally skin and bones, his muscles are stiff, his hearing is bad, and he has diabetes. But these limitations haven't slowed him down. He's a competitive professional cyclist. In 2011, he won the British National Para-Cycling Circuit Race Championship in his class. Not so bad.

While taking a break from some research, I read about Tom in an article on the BBC website. I was surprised to find that this genetically skinny man has type 2 diabetes—a disease that mostly affects overweight people. How could this skinny cyclist get diabetes?

It's no secret that eating too much sugar or too many carbs messes with your body's blood sugar balance. Blood glucose, which is basically sugar in the blood, is required for you to survive. Too little and you die. Too much and you risk getting type 2 diabetes.

When you eat sugar or carbs, your body produces insulin, a hormone that helps your body absorb sugar from the blood and store it in your liver, muscles, and fat tissue. Too much sugar in the blood causes the pancreas to release a flood of insulin. When this occurs, two things happen. First, the body's fat-burning capacity is switched off, so it can burn sugar as fuel. And then, because there is so much insulin in your bloodstream, your body stores too much sugar (which it converts to fat) and the glucose levels in your blood drop too low. This means you'll need to eat more sugar to bring them back into balance. More sugar, more insulin, more fat, less blood sugar—it becomes a cycle. Type 2 diabetes comes along when your pancreas says *I'm through with this roller coaster,* gets tired, and slows production of insulin.

But what about those cultures that eat traditional diets that are high in carbs and *don't* suffer from an epidemic of diabetes like we do? In his famous China Study, described as "the most comprehensive study of nutrition ever conducted," T. Colin Campbell, a researcher at Cornell University, found that while the rural Chinese diet is approximately 80 percent carbs and only 10 percent fat and 10 percent protein, it is extremely healthy for them.[1] They don't suffer from the high incidence of diabetes that urban-dwelling Chinese, who eat a more Westernized diet, do. If sugar or carbs were causing problems for the rural Chinese, they would be the largest consumers of insulin shots in the world, but they're not. So there must be another factor. What happens in Tom's body tells us what it is.

The other factor is fat—specifically, fat in the bloodstream.

Since Tom can't store fat, his blood is filled with it. His diabetes is caused by the excess fat in his blood, coupled with the normal amount of sugar and carbs in his diet. This is exactly what causes type 2 diabetes in most people—the combination of carbs and sugars with fat, not the sugar and carbs themselves. What this means is that a low-carb, higher-fat diet like the paleo will likely decrease your risk of diabetes just as much as a whole food, high-carb, low-fat diet will. The dietary combo that is the troublemaker is high fat plus high carb.

## Can Both Diets Work?

During my own weight-loss journey, still going on as I write, I've chosen to experiment with a high-vegetable, medium-protein, and lower-carb, lower-sugar diet. I've not entirely given up carbs and sugar. I'll eat some sugar from fruit with my smoothie every morning and will have some sort of carbohydrate, generally rice, at lunch or dinner. Good news is, I'm still losing weight. It's June, and I'm about 25 pounds down. I was down a few more, but I've been traveling for two weeks straight and have another two weeks of travel ahead of me. That's often when I gain a few pounds, though I lose them when I get home.

The diet I'm eating this time around seems to be the most comfortable for me. Nicholas Gonzalez, a holistic cancer doctor in New York City, once told me that he has a complicated process to determine the type of diet that works best for his patients. It includes a questionnaire, a consultation, and some blood testing to figure out what percentage of protein, fat, and carbohydrates they should be eating during their treatment. But ultimately, he says, if he just asks patients whether they like protein, their answer will, with surprising accuracy, match the full analysis of his testing.

Dr. Gonzalez is saying that there's no one-size-fits-all, low-carb or high-carb diet for healing people with cancer, so it's not much of a stretch to say that there's no one-size-fits-all carb diet for the rest of us either. How both low-carb and high-carb diets respond to diabetes should be enough to convince you that the side-taking on carbs is mostly based on dogma, not hard evidence.

Take the work of Neal Barnard, a leading clinical researcher who looks at the effects of diet on health. In a now-famous study published in 2006,[2] he found that a low-fat, high-carb vegan diet was more beneficial for treating diabetes than the diet recommended by the American Diabetes Association (ADA). After 22 weeks, 26 percent of those on the ADA diet, which recommended 15 to 20 percent animal protein and 60 to 70 percent carbohydrates, were able to reduce their diabetes medication. But of those who followed the low-fat vegan diet, 46 percent experienced the same results.

That said, the argument on the other side is equally convincing. A 2011 study at the University of California San Francisco (UCSF)[3] had a group of type 2 diabetics follow the Mediterranean diet, while another group tried the paleo diet. Within two weeks, those on the paleo diet had lowered their blood sugar, blood pressure, and cholesterol, while the diabetics on the Mediterranean diet experienced no improvements. The reason both the Barnard diet and the UCSF paleo diet work, at least for diabetics, is that they're both whole-food diets—that is, with no processed foods—and neither combines high fat with high carbohydrates.

To prove that my high-fat, high-carb theory isn't theory at all, you don't have to look much further than a 2011 study[4] conducted by researchers from the University of California and Sanford-Burnham Medical Research Institute that showed how a high-fat diet can pave the way for type 2 diabetes. With mice as their subjects, the scientists found that a high-fat diet increased fatty acids in the blood, hampering the development of the crucial enzyme GnT-4a, which helps regulate blood sugar. Combining a high-fat diet with high sugar intake throws blood sugar levels all out of whack, creating the optimal conditions for type 2 diabetes.

All this data is liberating. Essentially, it means you have some flex-ibility with the diet you can choose and still stay healthy. If you're doing the paleo diet for health reasons but you don't like meat, then switching to a low-fat, high-carb diet might be your thing. If you're a vegan for health reasons but love pulled pork more than quinoa cakes, a low-carb diet might be just as beneficial for you.

So yes, you can eat carbs and sugar from whole food sources, pro-vided you choose a high-carb, low-fat diet. If you choose a low-carb, higher-fat diet, you should eat fewer carbs and less sugar. And again, you should never eat a high-fat, high-carb, high-sugar diet.

### He Has His Cake, But Did He Eat It Too?

It's July 12, 2014, and we're celebrating Hudson's second birthday in our backyard with 20 or so of our friends and their kids. Annmarie brings out a car-shaped carrot cake made with gluten-free flour and sweetened with honey. The wheels are slices of kiwi fruit, and the icing is made with cream cheese and confectioners' sugar. Yes, that's right, processed white sugar.

At this point you can condemn me as a fraud if you like. But as a health writer who knows a lot of health experts and gurus, I'll tell you that the only difference between them and me is that I'm willing to admit that we baked a cake with white sugar icing. They'll make the cake but won't let you know about it.

So yes, sugar and processed carbs like white pasta and Ital-ian bread can be eaten as a treat now and then. But if you're a self-professed sugar addict or carb-oholic, I definitely recom-mend staying away from these foods. Sugar is highly addictive. In fact, Mark Hyman directed me to a study by Harvard researchers Belinda Lennerz and David Ludwig[5] showing how the brain re-sponds to sugar. They gave a group of overweight men two types of milkshakes: one shake contained a tasteless starch that spiked blood sugar quickly, while the other did not. Functional brain im-aging after drinking the shakes turned up clear differences: the sugar-spike shakes increased activity in an area of the brain "that's ground zero for addiction," as Mark Hyman put it, adding, "When you keep hitting that area of pleasure, you're going to keep wanting to hit it over and over and over again."

### I JUST NEED MY SWEETENER!

So you need your daily sweetener and don't want to put white sugar in your coffee. Here are some alternative sweeteners you could try:

**Stevia.** You'll never have to complain about stevia not being sweet enough. Made from the South American stevia plant, it's 200 to 300 times sweeter than sugar. Best of all, it has no calories, no carbohydrates, and no impact on blood sugar. Be sure to stay away from overly processed stevia, however, as it tends to have additives you don't want. The real stuff will be a green powder, not white.

**Lakanto.** This is a mix of the sugar alcohol erythritol and an extract from *luo han guo,* a Chinese fruit. Be mindful of the brand you use, since some erythritol is made from genetically modified corn.

**Xylitol.** Another sugar alcohol with an odd name, xylitol is found in the fiber of many fruits and vegetables, as well as in oats, mushrooms, and cornhusks. It gives you the sweetness you crave but with 40 percent fewer calories. It is heavily processed, however, so watch how much you use; too much can give you an upset stomach.

**Honey.** The oldest sweetener in the world, honey is hard to beat. However, you don't want just any old brand from the supermarket; some commercial honey comes from bees fed high-fructose corn syrup. Stick with organic brands, and if possible buy honey made by local beekeepers.

> **Maple syrup.** This is another natural sweetener. Be sure to get natural maple syrup, not those fake syrups labeled "maple flavored." Grade A syrup, the lighter variety, comes from sap extracted early in the season. It has a more delicate flavor than Grade B syrup, the darker variety. Made from sap extracted later in the season, Grade B syrup has an intense flavor and is best for baking.

If you have a sweet tooth, you might want to choose a lower-carb diet, so you won't be tempted to overeat that object of your abominable cravings. Nutritionist and bestselling author JJ Virgin agrees. Her Sugar Impact Diet is designed to bust through these cravings, which she says are both physiological and emotional. She withdraws people gradually over a two-week period, re-acclimating their taste buds to just how sweet sugary foods are. "You retrain your sweet tooth so you'll never want sugar again," she says. After that, you can introduce sugar back into your diet using medium sugar-impact foods like cherries, apples, sweet potatoes, watermelon, and brown rice.

### Gluten: Nutrition's Most Wanted

After Hudson's birthday cake is long gone and we're cleaning up. I notice that the pasta salad one of our friends brought is untouched. I wonder why. I take a bite. It's delicious, made with gluten-free quinoa pasta. It puzzles me why no one else ate it since it looked and tasted so good. But as I carry it to the kitchen, I realize why: no one knew it was gluten-free.

Gluten seems to be nutrition public enemy #1 these days. It would be irresponsible for me to talk about sugar and carbs and not mention the plant protein that causes more fear in the food obsessed than global warming and threat of global financial collapse combined.

A few weeks after the birthday party, following a guys' night of craft beer at Jupiter, a brewery in Berkeley, I wake up with a serious stomachache. On my way to the bathroom, I look in the mirror and find that my entire face is swollen. My eyes look like someone inflated the lids while I was sleeping, leaving me in a semi-squint. It's obvious that something in my smoked porter has caused a serious histamine reaction, along with the stomach wrench. Fortunately, I'm pretty sure I know what it is: the gluten in the beer. Unfortunately, this means I'm probably going to have to temper my love for malted barley and hops.

## Gluten Sensitivity: 12,000 Years New

A compound of the proteins glutenin and gliadin, found in wheat, barley, and rye, gluten is what makes bread rise and gives it a chewy texture. Though demonized now, gluten is in no way new to our diets. John Hawks, an anthropologist at the University of Wisconsin, says celiac disease, the most extreme kind of gluten sensitivity, is a "recent development" in human history, but by recent he means it developed 10,000 or so years ago, when wheat was first cultivated in the Middle East. While there's little evidence of celiac disease from way back then, there is some from the second century, when a noted Greek physician, Aretaeus the Cappadocian, described a stomach condition that left his patient tired, frail, and suffering with diarrhea, though he didn't associate it with wheat or gluten. British physician Samuel Dee dubbed the condition "coeliac affection," in an 1888 report since characterized as "the most vivid and accurate description of the clinical state which we still call coeliac disease."[6] But it wasn't until the 1950s that a strong association between celiac disease and gluten was noted.[7]

Now defined as an autoimmune disease caused by gluten, celiac disease is diagnosed quite consistently by functional medicine doctors, nutritionists, and even some conventional doctors. The same symptoms in a milder form are described as gluten intolerance or sensitivity.

Celiac disease affects only one percent of the population. But why is it that more people than ever before seem to have some form of gluten sensitivity?

## Is Gluten Sensitivity Really Exploding?

Many researchers tie the increase in gluten sensitivity to the hybridization of wheat in the middle of the 20th century. Plant scientist Norman Borlaug won a Nobel Peace Prize for spawning the so-called Green Revolution aimed at eliminating famine. But the hybridized wheat he re-engineered to increase yield and create a hardier plant also contained more gluten.

"Originally, I thought there was more celiac because we were better at finding it,"[8] Joseph Murray, a gastroenterologist and professor of medicine at the Mayo Clinic, said. But he was mistaken. For a study published in the journal *Gastroenterology* in 2009,[9] Murray's team compared blood samples collected from U.S. airmen between 1948 and 1954 with a sample from young men in the 2000s. The latter were four and a half times more likely to have celiac disease than their forebears.

## Why Is Wheat Gluten Bad?

Tom O'Bryan, or Dr. Tom to most, is a functional medicine doctor who started his practice over 30 years ago. He discovered the negative effects of gluten when his wife was trying to get pregnant and couldn't. So he called on seven of the best-known functional medicine doctors to help him out, and in six weeks his wife was pregnant. Then his neighbors, who were having the same problem, asked Dr. Tom how they'd done it, and in three months they, too, were expecting a child. Dr. Tom started using the protocol for all his patients, not just those trying to conceive, and achieved results for all sorts of conditions. One of the major factors in the positive results, he tells me, is that in all cases, he told his patients to get off wheat.

Ever since then, he's been on a mission to spread the news about just how much gluten can seriously mess up your health. He likens gluten to gasoline: it's the fire starter for autoimmune disease and inflammation. "All degenerative diseases at the cellular level are always inflammatory: diabetes, Alzheimer's, cardiovascular disease, arthritic disease, autoimmune diseases," Dr. Tom says. "So the key is an anti-inflammatory lifestyle, which means putting the fire out." Although sometimes heavy metals or toxic chemical exposure or imbalances were implicated in the conditions his patients suffered, food sensitivities were the most prevalent fuel, he found, gluten sensitivity above all.

One reason gluten is such a problem is that it's notoriously difficult to digest. On the Protein Digestibility Corrected Amino Acid Score (PDCAAS), where 1.0 is the most easily digested, whole wheat comes in at 0.42 and wheat gluten is an anemic 0.25, compared to 0.92 for beef and 0.78 for chickpeas.[10] When we can't break the gluten down into amino acids, we're left with clumps of undigested protein. If they get into the bloodstream, they cause an immune reaction. Inflammation from wheat gluten insensitivity leads to system-wide issues that include virtually all autoimmune disorders, from rheumatoid arthritis, fibromyalgia, and chronic fatigue to diseases of the thyroid and the adrenal glands.

### Is Everyone Gluten Sensitive?

Peter Osborn, a chiropractor from Sugarland, Texas, who specializes in gluten sensitivities, wants us all to become gluten-free warriors against what he sees as a hybridized gluten invasion. Early in his career, in the rheumatology department of a VA hospital, Peter saw many patients with "incurable" autoimmune diseases like rheumatoid arthritis, lupus, and the connective-tissue disorders scleroderma and dermatomyositis. When conventional treatments like medications only lessened symptoms, he took it upon himself to research what might cure these diseases. When Peter suggested putting some of the patients on a gluten-free diet, his superiors said no: they didn't think nutrition had anything to do with these conditions. Eventually, Peter left the hospital and went into practice on his own.

He tested his theory on one of his very first patients, a five-year-old boy who had been given six months to live after a diagnosis of juvenile rheumatoid arthritis. The Make-A-Wish Foundation granted the boy's wish, sending his entire family to the Galapagos Islands. But after Peter removed gluten from the child's diet, he started to heal. Now he's 15, healthy, and playing in his high school band.

According to Peter, gluten sensitivity is all-or-nothing. "It's kind of like being pregnant," he says. "There's no scale for it. You either are or you aren't." But how many of us actually are gluten sensitive? Peter puts the estimate at 40 percent. To find out if you're in that 40 percent, there's a genetic test, but you can also just pay attention to how your body reacts when you eat gluten. Better yet, see how your body reacts when you take foods made of wheat, barley, and rye out of your diet.

## IT MIGHT NOT BE GLUTEN: FODMAPS

Not everyone agrees that gluten is the devil—or the only one, at least. Peter Gibson and Jessica Biesiekierski, researchers responsible for a 2011 study[11] that helped popularize the gluten-free diet, did a follow-up study in 2013[12] in which they found that some of the gastrointestinal disorders attributed to non-celiac gluten sensitivity, aka gluten intolerance, may have nothing to do with gluten at all. The likely culprits, the study suggests, are FODMAPs, a group of short-chain carbohydrates and sugar alcohols, including fructose, lactose, oligosaccharides, and polyols, that are poorly absorbed in the small intestine; readily ferment in the colon, causing gas; and have a laxative effect. FODMAPs are found in a wide range of foods, many of which do not contain gluten, including garlic, onions, cruciferous vegetables, mushrooms, apples, pears, avocados, watermelon, honey, and dairy products, and in artificial sweeteners like sorbitol.

### A Compromised Warrior

I'm positive—gluten sensitive, that is. Because I'm writing this book, I got the genetic test Peter Osborn mentioned. I'm not happy to find out that I tested positive, though I'm not surprised. I already suspected that wheat is an issue for me, and judging by my reaction to the beer that night at Jupiter, I have antibodies to the proteins. My immune system is already engaged in the war against gluten.

While I'd like to think that Dr. Tom and Peter Osborn are extremists about gluten, I also know the ill effects of a weakened immune system and inflammation. I'm now a warrior who needs to take a side. So I decide to go gluten-free. I pretty much was before my last two years of gluttony, so going back isn't that much of a stretch. For me, the best way to avoid gluten is to keep wheat out of the house. I don't look for it when it isn't there.

What I'm not going to do is dig into absolutely everything I ingest to uncover hidden gluten. (It's even found in some toothpaste, though many popular brands are now gluten-free.) I won't completely give up beer right now, though I'll drink it much less often. I guess you could say that I'm a gluten warrior but also a spy.

## A Better Choice

The next time I'm out with friends, I order a glass of chardonnay with their first round of beers. They give me a hard time, but I simply shrug it off. They don't have to look at my marshmallow face in the mirror tomorrow. I also rib them a bit, telling them that since there are five of us at the table, odds are that there is one person in addition to me who's genetically inclined to gluten sensitivity and might wake up bloated tomorrow.

After a little more back and forth, one friend, sensing he has me cornered, asks, "If you're so concerned about your health, why are you drinking alcohol anyway?"

Unfortunately for him, he had no idea I had a pretty detailed comeback to that comment, too.

"Okay, so let me tell you a little bit about alcohol . . . "

# CHAPTER 10

# AN INTERESTING CONCLUSION ABOUT BEER, WINE, AND SPIRITS

"I'll meet you on the beach in 20 minutes for sunset," James tells me over the phone before we hang up.

Annmarie and I have just arrived in Sarasota for our annual check-up with him, and we're staying at a tiny RV park near the southern tip of Fiesta Key. It's the middle of winter, but it's 75 degrees here. The Gulf of Mexico is a 100-foot walk from our rig, so we head down early, find a picnic bench, and sit facing the water.

James arrives on time with a bottle of red wine, three glasses, and a *mapacho* cigarette. Mapacho is a tobacco smoked by shamans in the rainforest. The wine, James says, is from Sardinia. It's high in poly-phenols—antioxidants—and lower in alcohol content than California wines. He opens it and pours three glasses, then lights the cigarette and blows the smoke over the glasses as a blessing.

It's January 2011, six months before my three-minute wine-guz-zling experience with Sebastian at his home in Tica Tica, Peru. But at this point, I haven't had a sip of alcohol in nine years. I gave it up shortly after college because I didn't want drinking to define me. I was drinking too much and needed to grow up, find a purpose. At the same time, I was getting really serious about my health, so alcohol just didn't have a place in my life anymore. But now, almost a decade later, I'm different—confident but humble and on a path to find more balance. James has already convinced me that extremes aren't neces-sary for great health or a great life, so as I watch him sipping the red wine, I think maybe my extreme stance on alcohol has been wrong as well. Plus, I'm intrigued about the Sardinians after reading about them in *The Blue Zones.* Their long life includes wine, and secretly, I want mine to as well.

James hands the glasses to Annmarie and me, then dips his finger into his glass and flicks a drop of wine to the earth as an offering—just as Sebastian did in Peru. Annmarie and I repeat the gesture. I look to her with a shoulder shrug. She smiles back and nods with approval. I take a sip. I can't think of a better time and place to start this new chapter of experimentation than now, while the sun slowly sinks toward the ocean, pulling the strong blues out of the day and uncovering the warm hues of twilight.

James passes the cigarette to me. I grin and decline it. One vice at a time, I joke.

### Why Sardinians Don't Die of Cirrhosis

The Sardinian people both drink and live long. They drink a wine made from Cannonau, or Grenache, grapes with lunch and dinner. You'll sometimes see the wine labeled Cannonau di Sardegna or Cannonau followed by the name of a region within Sardinia. The Sardinians' daily, moderate imbibing doesn't seem to cause cancers of the mouth and esophagus, or any other illness associated with alcohol use, so what's their secret?

Some experts believe the reason why the Sardinians' alcohol consumption doesn't adversely affect aging and disease is because the Cannonau wine has two to three times the amount of flavonoids of other red wines, but I think these experts are being shortsighted. Flavonoids, the largest family of polyphenolic compounds, confer a wide array of benefits, having been shown to stave off everything from cancer to heart disease, but when you look more closely at the amount of polyphenols in Sardinian wine, it is, at best, average. If you have a glass of non-Cannonau grape wine and eat more than half a cup of blueberries, you'll get nearly double the amount of flavonoids you would get from a glass of this Sardinian staple.[1]

Additionally, you don't even need to look away from the Blue Zones to find a counterpoint. The preferred drink of the Okinawans is sake, which unless it's the kind that contains mugwort, or worm-wood, has much less polyphenol activity than wine. The Okinawans live pretty long, too. But whether you're drinking wine from cannonau grapes, or sake with or without mugwort, it's hard to believe that the flavonoids are what transmute the alcohol from innocent to harmful.

Let's be real. Every additional longevity-producing activity the Blue Zone cultures engage in besides drink—like walk all day long, spend time with extended family, live in community, eat a primar-ily plant-based diet, and enjoy relatively low stress—cancels out any negative effects of the alcohol.

Unfortunately, though, we're not all lucky enough to live on beau-tiful, isolated islands. I can only hope to break even longevity-wise when I drink, given that I'm sitting at a computer all day, stressing out about a book deadline, worrying about what school to put Hudson into, living 3,000 miles from my family, and eating dinner at the local farm-to-table BBQ smokehouse.

It seems, then, that for us non–Blue Zoners, there's a place for drinking, somewhere between teetotaling and downing pints like the guy at the end of the bar who's been there since it opened at 11 A.M. In fact, some science holds that those who drink live longer than those who don't. That may sound contradictory, since alcohol is toxic to the body, but it's hard to argue with some of the research.

A study published by Wageningen University in the Netherlands in 2009[2] that analyzed the health of a group of middle-aged men between 1960 and 2000 came up with some surprising results that should make you feel less guilty about having a glass of wine every day. Although the researchers were careful to point out that further studies were necessary, they found that long-term, light alcohol con-sumption was associated with increased life expectancy—five years more than nondrinkers could look forward to, in fact.

According to the Nutrition Source, an online service of Harvard's School of Public Health, more than 100 studies show that moderate drinking reduces the risk of heart attacks, strokes, and death from all cardiovascular disorders by 20 to 40 percent.[3] This seems to be ac-knowledgment that even for people who are not the longest lived in the world, alcohol consumption in moderation can be beneficial. But what is moderation? Unfortunately, this isn't as neat as a shot of Glen-fiddich either. What's considered moderate differs between countries and cultures, as well as in personal and scientific opinion.

## PROOF THAT ALCOHOL CAN BE HEALTHY

**It increases longevity.** A ten-year study in Japan[4] found that men and women age 40 to 79 who consumed one to two alcoholic drinks per day decreased their risk of mortality by 12 to 20 percent.

**It lowers the risk of death from cardiovascular disease.** A study of more than 36,000 middle-aged men in Eastern France[5] found that moderate consumption of wine decreased mortality risk from all causes, while moderate consumption of both beer and wine lowered risk of death from cardiovascular disease.

**It reduces the risk of Alzheimer's and dementia.** Researchers at Loyola University Chicago Stritch School of Medicine[6] reviewed studies covering more than 365,000 participants and found that moderate drinkers were 23 percent less likely to develop Alzheimer's disease or other forms of dementia.

**It increases good cholesterol.** Researchers at the University of Alabama at Birmingham[7] found that moderate intake of alcohol increased levels of HDL, the "good" cholesterol that helps stave off heart disease.

**It may protect against Helicobacter pylori.** A study at the University of Belfast[8] in Ireland shows that moderate consumption of beer or wine can protect the stomach against the H. pylori bacteria, which can cause ulcers, gastritis, and stomach cancer.

## A Bottle of Wine a Day?

If you dig through the data on alcohol, you find that moderation is a slippery thing to grasp. The National Institute on Alcohol Abuse and Alcoholism—part of the National Institutes of Health—defines "low-risk" drinking as up to four drinks per day for men, three for women, with a weekly limit of 14 drinks for men and 7 for women.[9] On the more conservative side, the Mayo Clinic in Rochester, Minnesota, says the limit for healthy adults should be one drink a day for women of all ages and men over 65, and two drinks a day for men age 65 and younger.[10]

At the other extreme is the amount endorsed by former World Health Organization (WHO) alcohol expert Kari Poikolainen, author of *Perfect Drinking and Its Enemies.* Poikolainen, a physician and adjunct professor of public health at Finland's University of Helsinki, drew a flood of criticism[11] after telling the *Daily Mail* that based on "decades of research" on the effects of alcohol, he concluded "that drinking only becomes harmful when people consume more than around 13 units a day."[12] To put that in perspective, a bottle of wine contains about 9 or 10 units of alcohol.

So somewhere between a glass and a bottle or so, we have moderation. But it's entirely possible that moderation isn't the only factor we should consider. Just as we're not Neanderthals anymore, most wine, beer, and spirits that we buy in the supermarket or liquor store are not what they used to be either.

I didn't realize this could be a factor in determining a definition of moderation until I learned about a rogue group of vintners in Northern California who are making wine the way wine is supposed to be made. They're nonconformists, doing stuff that other wineries would scoff at. They're environmentalists—but capitalists, too. They know that fine wine grown sustainably and biodynamically is not only good for the earth and good for you, but it's good for the bottom line as well.

John Williams is one of them.

## IT'S NOT ALL A PARTY:
## BOOZE AND YOUR WAISTLINE

Don't forget that alcohol is rich in calories. Even an ounce of vodka—mostly water and ethanol—is close to 100 calories, about the same as half a cup of ice cream. A 12-ounce bottle of beer with a 5 percent alcohol content contains 150 calories. And the same bottle filled with a stronger brew, such as Sierra Nevada Bigfoot (9.6 percent alcohol), contains a whopping 330 calories; two of those and you've just taken in more calories than a McDonald's Big Mac (550 calories). One small glass of wine (five ounces) filled with California cabernet sauvignon contains 145 calories.

However, alcohol content is what matters most in the calorie wars. Some German Rieslings contain as little as 8 or 9 percent alcohol, while certain Australian wines can top 16 percent. As a rule of thumb, wines from colder regions (Champagne, Loire Valley, Washington, Oregon) tend to contain less alcohol than wines from warmer regions, like Australia and California. A five-ounce glass of champagne can have as little as 120 calories for brut but as much as 175 calories for sweeter kinds.

Alcohol is not converted to fat by your body, but it's so rich in calories that the body immediately uses it as a source of energy, instead of burning fat from your food or your body's stores. When your body has plenty of alcohol to burn, it will store fatty acids in foods as body fat, so there's almost no chance you'll start burning your own body fat and lose weight.

When you're thinking about moderation, consider the effects of weight gain that may come with drinking. If you consumed a bottle of Pinot Noir a day, thinking it was healthy, you'd be adding 4,200 calories a week to your diet. Compare that to 3,500 calories—roughly the number of calories in one pound of body fat.

## Wine Isn't Always Wine

As we walk between a row of grapevines with John, the owner of Frog's Leap Winery in Rutherford, California, I notice that the soil feels pillow-like underfoot. With each step, my foot sinks in at least an inch. This is not your typical hard, dusty Napa Valley terrain. There's very little rain in this area from April to November, and right now it's July.

"Healthy soil, healthy vine, healthy grape, healthy wine," John tells Annmarie and me. "The very concept behind great wine is this idea that the grapes and the wine take the character, the soul, the flavor, from the soil into the vine. Every molecule in that grape, every molecule in that wine will be deeply connected to the soil it came from." This is called *terroir*, a French word loosely defined as the way the entire ecosystem influences the crop. I guess you could say it's a step further than our modern-day notion of organic, which allows corners to be cut just to get certification.

The soil here, John explains, is "filled with life and everything the vine needs to provide great grapes with deep flavor." In all but a handful of other wineries in Napa, we'd find hard, dry dirt between the vines. This, he says, is a product of shortsighted farming, of not paying attention.

It's clear that here at Frog's Leap, they do pay attention. One thing that's different about the way John farms is that his vineyard doesn't use irrigation. This is called dry farming and is essentially the traditional way of growing grapevines. All Napa Valley wineries used to dry-farm until the late 1970s and early 1980s. Now, nearly all the wineries use irrigation and feed their vines with chemical fertilizers in the drip.

John believes this switch in practices is similar to the rise of junk food consumption in America and around the globe. In fact, you would almost think that his talk about grapes could apply to people. He's more like a naturopath for his vines than anything else. Feeding a vine just water and nitrogen fertilizer from a drip irrigation system is like "feeding your kid sodas and a candy bars," he says, as we move from the vines into a well-kept vegetable garden on the property. Grapevines naturally grow their roots deep into the earth, but if you irrigate them, the roots stay near the top of the soil, where there is more disease.

John compares conventionally grown vines to people: "Let's think about our own health. If everyone is overweight and not exercising and eating junk food all the time, viruses pass like wild fire in that community. In a healthy community they would go much more slowly. It's the same in a vineyard," he says. "Almost all of our problems are dealing with issues that come from other farms."

Healthy vines also live longer. John explains that most conventional wineries have to replant their vines every 15 years or so. Dry-farmed vines like his have a lifespan of 100 to 120 years, with the yield only beginning to slow after 60 or 70 years. Healthy vines also know the right time to ripen. Conventional vines have lost this wisdom.

We walk by some apple trees that grow in a small grove between two large plots of vines and next to a chicken coop. It's clear that this is a real farm, not a pretender. The race to bring big, bold, and flavorful wines to the public has confused farmers and their grapes, but most important it has changed the wine. "We've used to pick grapes at 22 and 23 percent sugar," John says. That's still the practice at his winery, but "now people are picking between 28 and 30 percent sugar," he says. As a result, the alcohol content in California wines has gone from 12 or 13 percent to as much as 16 percent or even higher. "Everyone wants to get a little buzz every now and then, right? But how about on a bottle instead of a sip." John calls today the "steroid era" of wine. Just as many American baseball players in the late 1980s and early 1990s were using steroids to beef up their muscles to improve their batting, growers now are rushing to beef up their wines to improve sales.

Sugar content of the grapes—measured in degrees Brix, named for the 19th-century German chemist who first measured the density of plant juices using a handheld instrument called a hydrometer—is one indicator of ripeness but far from the only one. Determining when to harvest grapes is as much art as science, with the winemaker using sight, smell, taste, and touch to gauge factors like acidity, color, flavor, and tannins (compounds that influence the dryness or "mouth feel" of a wine) of the grapes.

As we're walking back to go in and try some of the wines, John runs over a list of things that are done to conventional wines to manipulate them and correct the errors made in the growing process. None of them sound like they're good for our health. Mega Purple is a grape concentrate added to many low-to-medium-tier red wines to achieve uniform color, taste, and mouth feel. Oxygen is added to the barrel to age a wine faster by speeding up fermentation. And to balance the increased sugar in the wine and bring back the acidity that is missing from conventionally grown grapes, many winemakers add tartaric acid. "An acidulated wine tastes a little bit like Tang," John says.

Vegans especially won't like to learn that things like dried blood, egg whites, casein, and isinglass, a compound derived from fish swim bladders, are added to some wines to reduce haziness. (This process is sometimes necessary; even John does it from time to time, but he makes sure customers know.)

Most of these practices are avoidable with good farming, John believes. His grapes ripen at the right time and his vines are healthier. His wine has less alcohol, less sugar, and more nutrients, and it usually doesn't need to be manipulated. It's nothing like most of the big-name wines you'll see at the liquor store.

This is a hopeful sign. If I can drink a healthier, old-world-style wine from my own Northern California backyard, I'm all for it.

## So What Is the Best Alcohol to Drink?

As we sip a glass of sauvignon blanc in a private room in the Frog's Leap LEED-certified farmhouse, I don't know if I've been seduced by John's personality and knowledge, but this wine tastes really fantastic. Light, drinkable, not too fruity.

I ask John if he's heard of Cannonau wine, but he's not sure. I might not have pronounced it correctly: it's *Can-no-now*. What I want to know is if old-world wines in Europe are grown like his, not like most other California wines.

On that score, he has bad news. "California wines and French wines were very similar when California had its renaissance in the '70s. There was kind of an early generation of people who were emulating the French style of wines—balance, restraint, respect for *terroir*. Those are fundamental principles of classic wine making." All that changed when irrigation was introduced in the late 1970s, and Europe started emulating American wines.

But it's not all bad news. "There's a new generation of winemakers who are saying enough already and are stepping back a little bit," John says optimistically.

On the walk back to the car, Annmarie and I go back to the soft, pillowy soil under the grapevines to take some pictures. When I'm here I feel so much better about drinking wine than I ever have before. If I'm going to drink wine, I know that this wine not only has the flavor of the soil but also has the personality of the vintner himself. It would be foolish to think that *terroir* didn't include the stewards of the land as well.

But I do feel the need to put all this talk of drinking in perspective. I'm not trying to prove that wine or beer or spirits are healthier than kale or cherries. They're not. Any alcoholic beverage will have fewer nutrients per calorie than any health food. So while you could live on kale and cherries, I wouldn't recommend drinking your daily caloric allotment from alcohol and hoping you'll stay healthy. Alcohol isn't a health food. It's something some people choose to drink along with their healthy diet.

And there are those who can't drink alcohol at all, or choose not to, either because they are allergic to yeast or gluten, or have addiction problems, or are sensitive to sulfites. Sulfites—sulfur dioxide compounds—are added to wine to preserve it, a practice that dates back to Roman times. So if you are sensitive to sulfur, it would make sense to not drink wine. Even sulfite-free wine contains sulfur, since it occurs naturally in grapes.

## Beer's Not What It Used to Be, Either

While the craft beer industry is booming, the mainstream beer companies are no different from the big-name wine producers: they're cutting corners in production and adding things you'd never suspect—or want to ingest. The labeling requirements for these additives are so lax, you'll never see them on the label.

One common beer additive is high-fructose corn syrup, that ubiquitous substance that increases your appetite and can be toxic to your liver. A study published in *The American Journal of Clinical Nutrition* in 2004 linked the increased use of high-fructose corn syrup in drinks to our climbing obesity rate.[13]

Caramel coloring, used to give beer its rich golden-brown color, is the most commonly used coloring in food and beverages. In some cases, it's made by heating a sugar compound along with ammonium compounds, which produces 4-methylimidazole (4-MEI), found to cause cancer in mice and possibly in humans. California now requires a warning label if consuming a beverage would expose you to more than trace amounts of 4-MEI. But my vote would be to stick to craft beers, which don't use the coloring at all.

Propylene glycol, another common additive, is used to stabilize foam in beer. It's generally considered safe, but quite a few people are allergic to it, experiencing itchy, irritated skin and swelling.

Healthy drinking, then, depends on a number of factors. Since you're not going to get much agreement on what constitutes moderation, I'd take a conservative line of one to three drinks daily and keep an eye on your blood test results. If things start to get out of whack, I'd blame booze rather quickly and experiment with removing it. But if you know you can and will drink, make sure to choose something high quality.

As we drive away from Frog's Leap, Annmarie and I make it a point to look at the other vineyards to see if they irrigate. You can tell when they do because about 18 inches above ground you'll see a black tube running along each line of vines. In 30 or so minutes of driving from Rutherford to just north of Vallejo, we count just three dry farming plots like John's out of the hundreds we pass.

Seeing these conventional vineyards makes me think about another crop that has gotten a bad rap from those in the health world: coffee.

# CHAPTER 11

# WHAT AN ALMOST-90-DAY EXPERIMENT (BINGE) TAUGHT ME ABOUT AMERICA'S MOST POPULAR PICK-ME-UP

I love coffee. I love the taste. I love the smell. I love the sound of it brewing. I love the buzz. I love the energy that it gives me. I even love the fact that I love coffee. I guess you could say I'm an addict.

But times have changed.

It's May 2012, and I'm clean. I quit coffee almost ten years ago. Back then I started reading books on health and learned quickly that one thing health gurus hate just as much as white flour and hydrogenated oil is coffee. *It wrecks your adrenals. It's too acidic. Anything that addictive can't be good for you.* I believed all that, so I stopped drinking coffee. It hurt to give it up. I felt like I was losing a part of my being. My morning assistant.

Even now, a decade after the fact, I still have emotional nostalgia about coffee. It's similar to the feeling you might have about a short, intense romance that ended before anything could go wrong. I'd always thought that if I were to cross paths with coffee again at the right place and right time, I might be swept off my feet for a second time.

As I sit across from my friend at a Berkeley cafe, this is just what's happening. The waiter places a steaming cup of espresso in front of him.

I'm being seduced.

## The Temptation

"You like espresso?" my friend asks.

I've tried it only once at this point, so I tell him, "No, not really."

"You want to try this? It's one of the best."

I can smell it from across the table. It is flirting with me. The steam is curling seductively into the air. I want to justify why it would make sense for me to have a sip. I'm already eating my whatever-goes, farm-to-table diet. I've already gained 35 or so pounds. My energy sucks. How bad would it be to start drinking coffee again? It might give me a boost that I desperately need. Plus, I rationalize, when I was drinking coffee before, I wasn't drinking organic or fair-trade coffee, and I was adding all that sugar and cream. This would be an upgrade.

I was intrigued to discover that the people in the Nicoya Peninsula in Costa Rica, one of the Blue Zones, drink plenty of coffee and are still among the healthiest, longest-lived people in the world. But the truth is, I don't need an excuse. I just *want* to try coffee again. If so many other people in the world drink coffee, why shouldn't I? And if I get hooked again, so what? I've already quit once. How hard would it be to quit a second time?

"Yes," I say, "I'll try it."

And I do. And it is good. Really good.

And so begins the somewhat loosely controlled 90-day coffee-drinking experiment (more appropriately, binge) that I have been curious to start for quite some time but feared would send me back into hopeless, dizzying lust. But this time, my dream is that I'll fall in love on my own terms. I'll swoon but use my mind to stay in control. I'll write my story on my blog to let everyone know what happens after the time is up. Doing so will hold me accountable to myself, because I'll have hundreds of thousands of people to be accountable to online. It seems like the right thing to do.

It also seems like an excuse. Lip service aside, for the next 90 days, I'll get to drink coffee—the thing I love so much that I never wanted to give up in the first place.

## The Experiment

On the walk home from the cafe, feeling light and energized from that sip, I outline my plan.

Every experiment needs a premise. Mine is to determine two things about coffee. First, I want to know if there is a difference between the way my body reacts to the convenience-store coffee I was drinking before and the artisan coffees and espressos available now. The second—and more wildly self-interested—question is: Can I drink coffee and not have any ill effects, such as adrenal fatigue, jitters, or caffeine crash? My hypothesis—and potential dream come true—is that yes, it's entirely possible.

But this is a loosely organized study. One reason is that I have a vested interest in drinking coffee for the rest of my life, so I decide to design my coffee-drinking experiment in the same way most pharmaceutical companies design their trials—so it can't fail. It will be loosely controlled—mainly because I don't have that much control—and if done (sabotaged?) correctly, the results will be in my favor, justifying my continued coffee drinking without guilt or fear or shame.

So this is what I come up with: I'll drink coffee or espresso every day for 90 days and see what happens. There will be a sample group of one—me—and the control will be me the day before I started, when I wasn't drinking coffee. Throughout the experiment I'll take a regular index of my skin, hair, emotional state, and adrenals. And since my theory is that not all coffees are created equal, I'll drink only organic and fair-trade coffees.

In terms of monitoring my progress, I will stop this experiment if I experience any overt signs of the coffee being harmful to me: mood swings; changes in my skin, eyes, or hair; a feeling of adrenal stress. If I'm still doing fine after 90 days, I'll get a blood test to see if my adrenal blood markers are showing any signs of decline.

By the time I reach our apartment, I have a complete plan. I tell Annmarie about it.

Instantly, I can tell she's agitated. "You can't do that!" she snaps.

"Why?"

"Because I want to drink coffee again, too."

She's jealous. Unfortunately for her, coffee isn't advised for breast-feeding moms. I tell her that one day, after my experiment goes remarkably well and she's no longer feeding Hudson, we'll share plenty of cups together. This seems to calm her down.

But as I say this, my enthusiasm wanes a bit. I realize that she'll only be an enabler for me if I get hooked again.

## If They Drink It, Why Can't I?

I lied to you. I did break my coffee abstinence many years ago, but for only five days.

It is 2004. For our engagement getaway trip, I have found a deal on a short stay at an eco-lodge called Morgan's Rock on the Pacific Coast of Nicaragua. Annmarie and I are staying in a screened cabin on a hill. It's just a short walk down to a private cove.

On the first morning, a woman knocks on our door and softly says, "Wake up, wake up," in deeply accented English. Then we hear her walk away. I get out of bed, walk to the door, and open it. Just outside is a table with a tray containing a thermos and two coffee cups. I pour Annmarie a cup. She has always been able to have just one of something and leave it, unlike me, so I pass.

I watch her take the first sip. Her eyes open wide. "Whoa!" she says.

"Whoa, what? Whoa, good? Whoa, bad?"

"Whoa. This is really good coffee." She takes another sip.

I can't resist. My willpower is no match for Ann's enthusiasm. Within 30 seconds of saying no, I'm sipping my own cup, and we're both sitting in bed raving. It doesn't have any bite. It isn't acidic. It doesn't leave an aftertaste like most coffees do.

Even better, an hour or so later, we don't feel jittery. The energy it gives us is clean, and there's no crash. For the next four days, Annmarie and I drink one or two cups every day, eagerly waiting for our coffee angel to knock every morning.

We ask the hotel staff about the coffee and find out that it is shade-grown organic Nicaraguan coffee. We can tell they're proud of it. Why wouldn't they be? It can be argued that coffee, though it originated in Ethiopia, grows better in the high-altitude tropical areas of Central and South America. These countries produce some of the best coffee on Earth.

Nicaragua is new to the coffee game, however, as it was first brought there in the 1800s. And while that's quite some time ago, coffee has a rich tradition going back much farther.

Ethiopian legend holds that the coffee plant was first discovered accidentally in the 9th century by a shepherd named Kaldi. Kaldi was minding his goats one day when he noticed they were leaping about wildly after eating the berries of a certain tree. Tasting one of the berries, Kaldi soon found himself leaping about, too. Like most legends, it's probably fiction, but it does contain a kernel of truth. The jolt of energy that coffee provides—along with the bewitching taste—hastened its spread around the world, captivating people for centuries to come.

When coffee made its way to Europe in the 17th century, it was shunned by many as a wicked, satanic drink from the East. However, Pope Clement IV, tasting coffee to determine if it should be banned, became smitten with the brew and gave it a papal nod. Another legend? Maybe.

Americans made coffee their hot beverage of choice after the Boston Tea Party and revolutionary fervor drummed up a national distaste for tea. In the centuries thereafter, people all around the world became addicted to the stuff, as the Dutch and the British set up coffee plantations wherever they landed in South America and the Caribbean.

Clearly, coffee is deeply rooted in our history. What's not clear is if it's healthy for us to drink. One sign that it's healthy is the fact that the Nicoyans in Costa Rica regularly drink a few cups a day, and they're among the longest-lived people in the world. If these people can live to 100 on their high-octane brew, I'm convinced that the coffee argument is not a clear yes or no. My hunch is that what's more important is the kind of coffee you drink.

## Health Benefits or Negatives?

It's a week into my experiment, and there's nothing spectacular to report.

I drink an espresso shot in the morning and notice that the size of the shot varies greatly between coffee shops. Sometimes it seems small and accurately poured. Other times, I feel like I'm getting two or three shots for the price of one. On those days, I definitely get more of a wake-me-up. Overall, though, I have no jitters or ill effects from the espresso, and while I enjoy all the different flavor notes, I prefer the stronger, creamier-tasting pours to the sour ones. I've tried two small cups of coffee as well, but they did give me the jitters, so now I stay away.

I re-examine some research I did on coffee in the past and dig into some newer findings. The conclusions seem to be a muddled mess of nobody-can-agree. On the positive side, coffee consumption is linked to lowering the risk of many diseases, from diabetes to cancer. A study in Finland, which has one of the highest rates of coffee consumption in the world, tracked 14,000 men and women for a dozen years. It found that men who drank at least ten cups of coffee daily had a 55 percent lower chance of developing type 2 diabetes than those who drank two cups or fewer a day. For women, the difference was even more staggering. Those who drank ten or more cups a day had a 79 percent lower risk of developing diabetes than those who drank no more than two cups a day.[1]

A famous study that grew out of the Honolulu Heart Program, which tracked the health of 8,004 Japanese men for 30 years, found that the incidence of Parkinson's disease decreased among those who regularly consumed coffee. Those who drank the most coffee were least likely to get Parkinson's. The same effect was observed in those who consumed caffeine from other sources.[2]

A study conducted by the University of South Florida and the University of Miami and published in the *Journal of Alzheimer's Disease* in 2012 found that drinking two to three cups of coffee a day may help elderly people with memory problems delay the onset of Alzheimer's by two to four years.[3]

Researchers at Harvard Medical School found that women who consumed three cups of coffee a day were 21 percent less likely to develop skin cancer than those who drank only one cup a month. For men, the difference was 10 percent.[4]

The polyphenols found in coffee are credited with most of the benefit. Polyphenols are complex plant-derived antioxidants that protect us from disease by attacking free radicals, unstable molecules that cause illness and aging.

It's not all good news, though. On the negative side, coffee could be indicted on a few counts.

As many devoted coffee drinkers will attest, caffeine withdrawal can cause blazing headaches. Caffeine constricts blood vessels in the head, and once the input of caffeine stops, the blood vessels return to their normal size, abruptly increasing circulation in the brain.

Two substances in coffee, cafestol and kahweol, have been shown to increase cholesterol levels anywhere from 10 to 23 percent. And the acidity of coffee triggers everything from gastroesophageal reflux disease to ulcers. A 2001 study by a cardiologist at Henry Dunant Hospital in Athens, Greece, found that the amount of caffeine in just one cup of coffee is enough to harden arteries and increase blood pressure.[5]

But my question is: What kind of coffee was used in their studies? Does it make a difference?

### Yes, It's True: All Coffees Are *Not* the Same

The first time I met Dave Asprey was in May 2013. He spoke at a small, invite-only health industry event and throughout the day was wearing amber-tinted sunglasses in the conference room. I'm a little skeptical of people who wear sunglasses inside, so I didn't know what to think of him.

Silly me.

A week or so later, I found out that Dave's amber-tinted glasses weren't a fashion statement. They block blue light, which disrupts sleep and melatonin production. I had recently bought a pair myself. So I gave Dave a second shot.

Dave is a coffee evangelist. His passion isn't only selling his own carefully sourced beans; it also includes explaining just about everything that is wrong with most coffee in the grocery store.

Back in the 1990s, Dave, a self-proclaimed computer geek, started a technology career in Silicon Valley. Soon after, he found himself over 300 pounds and miserable. At the end of the decade, tired of how he felt, he started to research ways to get healthy. Some 16 years and $300,000 later, Dave is 100 pounds lighter and one of the best-known health- and bio-hackers on the planet—someone who uses technology as well as plain old prudent health advice to live an extraordinarily healthy life.

Somewhere along the line, Dave, like me, decided he wanted to figure out how to drink coffee, which he loves, and not get headaches. He found that certain coffees didn't leave his head pounding, and when he dug deeper, he uncovered the source of problems in coffee: mold toxins, pesticide contamination, and caffeine content.

"There are no health benefits to mold toxins," Dave points out. "From a long-term health perspective, avoiding as many toxins as possible is a good idea. Coffee is a high mold-toxin food, and most people who feel jittery, get headaches or sore joints, or feel like they can't tolerate coffee are not actually responding to coffee; they're responding to what else is in the coffee."

All agricultural products have some mold, he explains, and most countries have set limits on the amount of toxins that can be present in coffee. The United States and Canada, however, do not have restrictions on the most damaging toxins in coffee.

What mold toxins can do, Dave goes on to say, is trigger an autoimmune reaction: "Mold is directly toxic to your cells." An autoimmune reaction occurs when your immune system can't tell the difference between your good cells and these unhealthy invaders, so it just destroys everything it can. Essentially, your body goes to war with itself.

Conventional coffee with toxins in it also "has a stronger effect on the adrenals," Dave says. "Any time you ingest a toxin or something that causes a metabolic burden, it increases the stress on the body." One mold toxin in particular, ochratoxin A, is linked to cancer of the kidneys and bladder.

Just the thought of all these unregulated mold toxins in conventional coffee sends me on a Google search for brands that have low levels of mold. Dave's Bulletproof Coffee is one brand that does.

Pesticide residues are the second thing that should make you think twice about what brand you're buying. Coffee is generally heavily sprayed. Although the United States limits the kinds of pesticides that can be used in agriculture, such regulations don't exist in many of the countries we import our coffee from. Thankfully, there are an increasing number of certified organic import brands.

The third problem with coffee is the obvious one: caffeine. When we talk about coffee from a health perspective, we're really talking about caffeine, the chemical compound that gives you the buzz. What makes the issue even more confusing is that caffeine content varies widely with the bean and the brewing process.

Dave's brand, Bulletproof Coffee, has nearly half the caffeine content of coffee from other name-brand coffee bars. He had them tested. Dave cites "stressed plants" as one reason why some beans contain so much more caffeine than others. Caffeine acts as an antifungal agent in the coffee plant, he explains, and "the more stressed the plant is by fungus, insects, droughts, or nutrient deficiency, the more caffeine it makes."

Conventional coffees have more mold, so the plant produces more caffeine as a defense mechanism. Coffee lower in fungus is lower in caffeine. Coffee that's lower in caffeine is properly balanced, giving you the right amount of polyphenols and other health-giving nutrients with less of the compounds that can cause negative effects.

## DAVE'S RULES FOR COFFEE DRINKING

Dave, as you've probably figured out by now, is a coffee guru with a deity-like understanding of the brew. From this level of insight, he's handed down a few—well, five—commandments for appreciating this marvelous bean:

> **Never drink instant coffee.** It comes from cheap beans that tend to be moldier.
>
> **Try to drink coffees from Central America,** which are grown at high elevations, as they tend to be less contaminated by mold.
>
> **Stay away from decaf.** It, too, tends to be moldy.
>
> **Aim for wet-processed beans.** In wet processing, the fruit covering the bean is removed before it's dried. This method improves the consistency and cleanliness of the bean.
>
> **Avoid major brands,** as they tend to mix coffees from different growers, which allows for more contamination. Stick with smaller, single-estate coffees.

## Back to the Lab

Three weeks into my experiment, I decide to upgrade to a double shot of espresso every morning, because I want to up the caffeine and see how my body responds. One shot no longer gives me the buzz I'm craving when I wake up. I want to see if two can sustain it. They do. What I fail to see is that craving espresso and increasing my dosage are warning signs of addiction.

Over the next three weeks, I try drinking brewed and pour-over coffee to see if my body responds any differently from how it did before. Because I'm now habituated to more caffeine, I don't get jittery as long as I have only one cup. But even one cup makes my hands clammy 15 to 30 minutes after I drink it. This, for me, is a very clear sign of overtaxed adrenals.

Even Annmarie starts to notice changes. One morning she tells me that my eyes are bloodshot. I check for the next three days, and the whites are very red.

Finally, one morning, I get out of the shower and check my hair. It seems frizzier and more brittle than usual. I pass it off as the weather, but over the next few days the hair stays the same. Annmarie agrees that it looks dry and unhealthy.

The warning signs are adding up: craving, clammy hands, bloodshot eyes, dry and brittle hair.

## CAFFEINE BY THE CUP

You're not going to get the same amount of caffeine from a cup of green tea as you will from a shot of espresso. An energy drink will contain a bit more than a latte. Here's how the caffeine-delivery beverages stack up:[6]

8-ounce cup of coffee: 25 to 200 mg

8.46-ounce can of Red Bull: 80 mg

1-ounce espresso shot: 47 to 75 mg

8-ounce cup of black tea: 14 to 70 mg

8-ounce cup of green tea: 24 to 45 mg

## The Last Straw

Six weeks in, I realize that as much as I've stacked the deck to make this experiment go my way, the results are less than promising. Somewhere between week six and week seven, my fingers and hands start to hurt when I type. Not excruciating pain but enough to make me stop every ten minutes or so to exercise my fingers. Since I spend a good portion of my day at the computer, this symptom commands my attention. The hair, the eyes, the swampy hands, no big deal: I can live with them. But messing with my work is not something I can tolerate.

While I don't know exactly what is causing the pain in my hands, I know it's possible that it's linked to the findings of another Finnish study. After analyzing the medical records of some 25,000 people for just over 15 years, researchers found a strong link between the amount of coffee consumed daily and the likelihood of developing rheumatoid arthritis.[7]

I decide to quit my experiment early. But there's a problem: I'm hooked again.

### Quitting (Again)

I continue drinking coffee for another two or so weeks. On the symptom side, my hands are starting to hurt even more. On the emotional side, I've decided that since I know I'm going to quit eventually, I'll go all in. Typical addict behavior. I start drinking coffee all day long. A red-eye—a shot of espresso in a cup of regular coffee—in the morning, a pour-over at 11, an espresso at 2. Every day now I've got the jitters, I'm nauseous, and I'm agitated. Clearly I'm going out with a bang. Hitting rock bottom. Knowing this might be my last chance to drink coffee, I want to make sure I savor it.

You may roll your eyes when you hear caffeine described as a drug, but that's an accurate description. Back in 1994, the National Institute on Drug Abuse declared that caffeine was addictive in much the same way as alcohol and heroin. This is because caffeine has a structure similar to that of a molecule called adenosine, which is responsible for the tiredness we naturally feel as the day wears on.

Adenosine receptors in your brain can't tell the difference between adenosine and caffeine, allowing caffeine to slip into adenosine's parking space at those receptors. This creates a sense of alertness since adenosine is unable to do its job lulling you to sleep. This is fine right until the moment the effect of the caffeine wears off, allowing all that blocked adenosine to flood your receptors, creating the crash, the grogginess you hate so much. Most people deal with it by reaching for another cup. Once this goes on for a while, you sprout more adenosine receptors, which then require more caffeine to produce the alertness you're chasing. In time, especially for the more sensitive among us, this becomes an addiction.

I know I have to quit, but I also know weaning isn't going to work. I'm out of control. In my past work helping people change their diet and exercise habits, I've learned that the secret to lasting change is to replace the substance that is causing a problem with one that is almost as enjoyable but healthier. Eventually the body adapts, and you've created a new, healthier habit.

I choose green tea as my replacement. Now I just need to set the date of the swap.

I'm sure I could drink Dave's coffee or other well-sourced brands on a regular basis, but for me, quitting altogether is better than being tempted. This is strictly a personal decision. I encourage those of you who are able to drink coffee in moderation to try brands like Bulletproof or Food for the Mortals Organic Longevity Coffee, sourced by author and natural health and nutrition expert David Wolfe for his online store, Longevity Warehouse.

One morning—way after the quit date I'd set for myself—I wake up and make myself a cup of organic green tea. As I drink it, I want coffee, but I know that green tea is better for me.

On the walk to work, I notice a gentle buzz that feels nice. It's not the same caffeine punch that coffee gives me, but I don't feel jittery. The buzz wears off smoothly, and I don't crave more caffeine to keep me going or experience any withdrawal symptoms.

The next morning, green tea again. Same feeling, same results. This continues for the rest of the week. I'm gathering some momentum and excited that I'm moving on.

## We're All Different

My experiment was not a complete failure, though the results were disappointing. I did everything I could to make sure that it would turn out in my favor, but it didn't. Coffee and I just don't get along.

But I still wonder why I can't drink coffee, while some others can drink two cups at 10 P.M. and fall asleep 20 minutes later. Turns out, the reason is genetic.[8]

Essentially, there are two genes responsible for giving orders to produce the enzymes and nucleotides that determine how fast or slowly you metabolize caffeine. Fast processors can drink more coffee with fewer ill effects. Of the people tested by 23andMe, a genetic testing company, 51 percent are slow caffeine metabolizers.[9] The other 49 percent are lucky.

### Picking Up the Pieces (a New Coffee-Free Existence)

It takes about three or four days for my red eyes to clear up. My hair starts to get its shine back in a week, and by two weeks, my hands are no longer clammy and cold, and they've stopped aching.

This transition back to normal is fun to see. I usually don't see health results when I do things like take a new supplement or switch my diet a bit. Those changes are subtle. What I'm seeing now is evidence that the body knows what it needs and adjusts accordingly, as long as we keep it fueled correctly. My 90-day experiment confirmed that coffee is not for me. But you have to make your own decision about coffee, based on how you feel and how your body reacts.

Speaking of experimentation, this is perfect time to introduce you to the truth about another hotly contested food—salt. The next chapter of the story starts south of the border.

# CHAPTER 12

# SALT: NO GOOD FOR SLUGS, BUT WHAT ABOUT US?

"Where's the boat?" I ask John.

I'm riding shotgun in his Toyota RAV4, and we've just turned off the road and onto an unmarked sandy track, headed to the flats south of the lagoon outside Cuyutlán, Mexico. Cuyutlán is on the western coast, about four hours south of Puerto Vallarta and a two days' drive from Acapulco. On either side of the makeshift road are prickly pear cactus and other low, dust-coated brush.

"Huh? Who told you there was going to be a boat?" He laughs.

It was a good question. I had no idea. I just assumed the *sea* in sea salt meant there would be a floating vessel at some point during this trip.

"No boats here," John says, smirking. Annmarie would be happy to know this. She was adamant that I wear a life vest if I got on any boat.

John isn't your normal salt baron, if there even is such a thing. He's an ex-pat American surfer in his mid-40s who moved his family from Seattle to Sayulita, Mexico, a few years ago. Unlike other salt dealers in the area, John and his business partner, Geordie, who's in the back seat, weren't born into the salt business or descended from blue-collar Mexican laborers. John is a trained educator, a teacher. Geordie, originally from Bermuda, was at one time a hotshot firefighter for the U.S. Forest Service.

How they got into the salt business is more fortuitous than anything else. They discovered this salt when they moved to Sayulita and fell in love with it. But just because you find a good product—which they now call Aztec Sea Salt—doesn't mean you can turn around and sell it. They first needed to find out where it came from, and if that worked out, they'd need to find someone who would sell it to them. And then they needed to find a way to spread the message about it. Luckily, through a job working for a diet-book author, John had connections to people like me who love artisan salt and believe we need at least some of it to stay healthy.

Up ahead, we see an old beat-up truck limping toward us. If a truck could be a person, this one would be an old man without teeth or dentures; its entire front grille and hood are gone. As it approaches, we pull aside to let it pass. It's easily 18 to 20 feet long, and in the back, rising from behind the cab, are wooden racks struggling to hold what must be five or more tons of salt. The weight of the cargo pushes the racks outward, but surprisingly, the salt stays put. Over the next few minutes, we see five more of these trucks, all with distinct personalities and in various stages of decay, with the exception of one with two blown tires. The driver stands next to that truck, unconcerned. He waves happily at us.

Another quarter of a mile and John points to a few white mounds. "Almost there," he says. "You can see the piles of salt."

The reason I'm here is to see how salt is made . . . or harvested . . . or mined. I honestly have no idea which one it is. I also had no idea until about six months ago that some sea salt was produced in Mexico, but I was tipped off by a friend who told me about an amazing bag of salt he got from two ex-pats living on the western coast of Mexico just north of Puerto Vallarta.

I've come because I want to get to the bottom of the salt debate. There are a lot of health experts who would proclaim that their perspective on salt is so unwaveringly true that it may have been the lost 11th Commandment. But I don't care much for religious fervor when it comes to my health. What I want to find out is simply this: Is salt healthy for you? Does it cause stroke and high blood pressure, or is it essential for keeping our bodies functioning perfectly? I need to put the argument to rest for good. Visiting a place where salt has been harvested for more than a millennium seems like a good start.

## Salt Like Snow Piles

Before we go out on the flats, we stop in Cuyutlán. John explains that when the Mexican government shut down train service to this small coastal town, it got even sleepier than it is now. I don't see anyone on the streets. There are no cars. The only thing here, it seems, is salt—tons of it. Literally.

As we pull up to a salt depot—a collection of warehouses built out of wood from the palm trees—I see at least a dozen loading bays open to the street. Inside are mounds of salt that reach almost to the ceiling and extend the entire length of the building, maybe 100 feet. I've never seen this much salt in my life. It reminds me of the huge snow piles in the cul-de-sac where I grew up, after the snow plow came through during a rough Connecticut winter.

Salt is a 500-year-old industry in these parts and the only thing that has allowed the town to survive. This is just one of many examples of how salt and humans have coexisted for centuries. Salt has been part of the human diet for as long as there has been recorded history. Ever since worldwide trade began, salt has been one of the most valued commodities. The wealth of Venice in ancient times came largely from the salt trade. The Moorish merchants of the 6th century exchanged gold for salt. Salt was a valuable substance that could be used as currency.

Even in more civilized times, salt was a big deal, giving rise to revolt and shifting the entire history of some countries. Under the notorious reign of Louis XVI, the citizenry's dissatisfaction with the high salt tax in small part spawned the French Revolution. During the El Paso Salt War of the 1800s, American businessmen and Mexican citizens came into conflict over ownership of the Salt Flats in Mexico, nearly spawning a war between the two countries. Salt tax had the same effect in British-ruled India in the 1930s, inspiring Mahatma Gandhi and his followers to make their own salt at the seashore in protest. Salt's culinary use throughout history comes from its ability to enhance flavor and help preserve food in the absence of refrigeration.

The issue with salt, and why I believe the arguments for and against it are so polarizing, is that we do need some of it. But at both extremes—eating no salt and eating way too much—there is equal danger. If you don't have enough sodium (the Na from the NaCl), you die. On the other, more extreme hand, too much sodium will also kill you. You won't find many foods that have the same dire bounds as salt. Yes, you can eat too much corn or too much basil, but it's not going to make your heart stop. And if you don't eat enough of those things, no big deal. You won't croak from pesto deficiency.

And if you like getting clues from nature, like I do, think again. You won't find much there either. Deer will spend hours at a salt lick. My cat, Jonny 5, will shamelessly lick my sweaty arms. Slugs? Well, slugs hate salt for the very fact that it destroys them in seconds. So somewhere in between necessity, obsession, and instant death, there must be a place for salt in our diet, but where is it?

To find that place, I need to take a deep look at both extremes—too much and too little salt in the diet.

## Too Little Salt?

As we reach the salt farms, the land in front of us is dotted with carefully laid out rectangular patches of black trays filled with water. Ahead, by some of the harvesting areas, I see mounds of white salt. We stop by one that's seven or eight feet tall. There must be two or three tons of salt in the pile.

John gives me a tutorial on how the salt is harvested. Since there is no surface water in sight, he explains that the *salineros*—the salt farmers—dig down as much as ten meters or more into the brackish water table and pump the water up to the surface into the rectangle trays.

Once water is pumped into the trays, it sits there for one or two weeks. During that time, the salt farmers periodically scrape the bottom of the trays for sediment, adding more water as it evaporates.

The water in the trays becomes increasingly saline. Finally, once this salt water no longer has any more sediment and the saline content is right, the water is pumped into smaller, shallower trays. Twelve hours later, there is salt—piles of it. Eventually, the piles are dumped into a larger pile and then loaded into trucks and driven to town to be sold.

Seeing this process confirms that this salt is an artisan product, but just being artisan doesn't mean something is healthy. So while the process is interesting, the health implications are why I've come all this way to find out about salt.

The reason many health experts say we should eat salt (more specifically sodium) is that we need at least some of it to stay alive. The minimum daily requirement is around 500 milligrams of sodium, which is less than one-quarter teaspoon of salt There's even a name for not getting enough salt—hyponatremia, or "not enough salt in the blood." The symptoms of hyponatremia mimic those of dehydration, and if they're severe, can cause coma or death. This is largely a risk to those who participate in extreme activities. Long-distance runners are at the top of the list.

In 2003, the Department of Pathology at Massachusetts General Hospital assessed the sodium and hydration status of 140 collapsed runners in the medical tent at the 2003 Boston Marathon.[1] While most were dehydrated, 6 percent of them were hyponatremic. Most likely their sodium levels were so low from drinking too much water during the race, which upset the sodium-to-fluid ratio in their bodies so much that they fell ill from the imbalance.

The solution to hyponatremia, if the symptoms are not severe, is simply to add sodium—to stop drinking water and eat some salt. More serious cases might require a saline IV drip.

So, clearly we need sodium to stay alive, but what about to maintain health? Sodium is essential to the proper regulation of our bodily fluids. It allows us to sweat and balances the water inside and outside our cells. And in its interplay with aldosterone, a hormone secreted by the adrenal glands, sodium plays a crucial role in keeping our blood pressure from going too high or too low.

There are some health practitioners who challenge the long-held belief that too much salt is bad for you. Holistic physician David

Brownstein, author of *Salt Your Way to Health,* argues that a healthy diet with unrefined salt that hasn't been stripped of its original minerals can be beneficial for everything from blood pressure to fatigue.

Whether or not this claim is supportable, it's apparent that sodium is necessary to functional health. However, many anti-salt pundits will quickly catch me here and venomously explain that sodium doesn't have to come from table or sea salt. They are right about that. You can get sodium without eating salt. Fruits and vegetables contain it, and so does meat.

In the Dietary Guidelines for Americans provided by the U.S. Department of Health and Human Services, the maximum daily intake of sodium is 2,300 milligrams, just about a teaspoon of salt, since salt is approximately 40 percent sodium by weight. The recommended amount of sodium is even less: 1,500 milligrams, or less than three-quarters of a teaspoon. Most Americans consume quite a bit more sodium than the maximum recommended amount, upwards of 3,400 milligrams daily, or approximately one and a half teaspoons of salt.[2]

In order to get enough sodium, you could piece together a salt-free diet that would put you over the 500-milligram minimum, even up into the 1,500- to 2,300-milligram range. But this is just the type of neurotic health behavior that I want you and me to avoid. It's no fun keeping a spreadsheet of the sodium content of all the foods you eat in a week.

It's also not even necessary. While looking through the research about salt, I found evidence that points to a conclusion very different from the dominant view. What if I told you that you didn't have to worry about how much salt you ate, as long as you followed three simple rules?

The first simple salt rule is to not be foolish about your salt intake. Add it to your soup or marinate your veggies and meats with it, but don't go overboard. Use common sense.

The second rule is also simple: eat whole foods, because processed foods are high in added sodium. The rule may be simple, but the reasoning behind it is controversial. This is where the salt debate gets interesting.

One of the most popular recommendations from health authorities—it's handed out like strip-club flyers in Times Square—is to reduce your sodium intake. This recommendation comes largely from epidemiological research showing that people living in countries where sodium intake is high (even by American standards) tend to have higher blood pressure and more strokes.[3]

But this data doesn't always add up. Additional trials have found no correlation between salt intake and high blood pressure. The Intersalt study, the first large-scale look at salt use and blood pressure, published in 1988, confirmed a link between the two.[4] But critics later questioned the findings. True, the four populations with the lowest daily salt consumption also had the lowest incidence of high blood pressure. But these groups were outliers, from remote tribal and rural societies. Among the remaining 48 groups studied—all from the developed world—the link was hardly clear. Tianjin, China, which had the highest salt intake (about 14,000 milligrams a day, or 5,514 milligrams of sodium), had lower average blood pressure than Goodman, Mississippi, which had the lowest salt consumption (about 7,200 milligrams a day, or 2,836 milligrams of sodium).

In 2004, the Cochrane Collaboration, an international, independent, not-for-profit health care research organization funded in part by the U.S. Department of Health and Human Services, also found a lack of data connecting high blood pressure and salt consumption in 11 salt-reduction trials. Another review of 57 trials came to the same conclusion: low-salt diets don't yield substantial benefits over regular salt intake.[5]

Keep in mind, these results are statistical. That means there were some people in the studies who showed great improvement with reduced salt and others who showed none, or might even have gotten worse. It's also possible that people with hypertension—high blood pressure—could drop their blood pressure from 140/90 (the baseline for these clinical diagnoses) to 139/89. This is hardly encouraging, since they've made only a slug's worth of progress on the risk of stroke or heart disease. There's evidence that sticking to the recommended maximum sodium consumption for the day—2,300 milligrams—can make a slight difference in reducing high blood pressure. But the most dramatic impact comes from completely giving up added salt and consuming under 1,000 milligrams a day of sodium occurring naturally in food.

Studies like these cast doubt on the claim that salt is the only—or greatest—contributing factor to high blood pressure. What if the culprit is not salt but the quality of food people eat?

In a study of a modified Mediterranean diet called the DASH (Dietary Approaches to Stop Hypertension) diet, participants were fed fruits, vegetables, whole grains, low-fat meats, fish, and dairy with three levels of salt intake: low (2.9 grams a day), medium (5.8 grams a day), and high (8.7 grams a day). The control group ate a typical American high-sodium diet. The findings were impressive: The DASH diet, at all three levels of salt content from high to low, led to a significant reduction in blood pressure, compared to the control diet. The findings suggest that salt intake does lower blood pressure, but not a significant amount, and definitely not more than a healthy diet alone.[6]

All these findings fly in the face of salt recommendations we're normally fed. Even at 2,900 milligrams, which the American Heart Association and Health Canada and others say is still too much, a healthy diet like the DASH can lower blood pressure more than a diet restricted to 1,500 milligrams of sodium. This suggests that you can add more salt to your diet and still get healthier, as long as you maintain a whole-food diet. There's some evidence that this result is related to how insulin affects the kidneys.[7] Too much insulin inhibits your body's ability to excrete sodium. People who eat processed foods and excess sugar tend to produce too much insulin, which is probably why high blood pressure persists even with a reduced salt diet. The inability to excrete salt throws off the sodium-water balance in the body.

So, back to rule number two: eat whole foods. Whether salt intake is healthy or not is related to your entire diet, not just how much salt you consume.

And in case you're wondering about the connection between stroke and salt, the two major causes of stroke are blockages and ruptures in your blood vessels. Both lowering blood pressure and allowing your arteries to heal with a healthy diet will help reduce your risk.

Finally, the third simple salt rule is: quality matters. Here in Mexico, I've certainly found that.

John tells me that most table salts have been stripped down to one simple molecule—NaCl, sodium chloride. Back in the 1850s, older traditions of making salt gave way to increasingly mechanized processes, ushering in large-scale salt refining that strove for consistency. Removing so-called impurities, even if they gave salt its distinctive character, became the industry standard.

The next big shift came in the 1920s, when goiter, or iodine deficiency, became widespread. Salt manufacturers were persuaded to add iodine to table salt, a practice that continues to this day. Why choose salt to deliver the iodine? Think about it: it's the one food item consumed with nearly every meal. Furthermore, it doesn't spoil. Two recent studies consulted army records dating back 100 years to see what impact the iodization of salt had beyond halting the spread of goiter. One study suggested it led to a gradual increase in the IQ of U.S. males, while the other linked it to a gradual increase in the height of Swiss men.[8]

Iodine is an essential nutrient, but it occurs naturally in plenty of seafood, including shrimp, cod, and seaweed, as well as in yogurt, cheese, milk, and eggs. Eating a gram of table salt to get your recommended daily allowance of iodine seems like a poor nutritional choice.

Most health experts consider sea salt healthier than ordinary table salt. Standing next to a pile of it in Mexico, I'm tempted to say it's because of the mineral content; sea salt can include up to 92 different minerals. But after looking deeper into it, I learned that most of the trace minerals in sea salt have minimal benefit on your overall health. And you're better off getting essential minerals like potassium and magnesium from food, including fruits, leafy greens, nuts, and beans.

That said, I still strongly recommend sea salt. Most artisan sea salts have not been bleached or had calcium silicate added to them to prevent caking. Furthermore, most sea salts have better flavor and a much smoother mouth feel than table salt because of the broader spectrum of minerals. In all the discussion of health, we forget that we salt food to make it taste better.

There are well over a hundred sea salts available these days, many of them artisan. Check the shelves of any gourmet market or online. John sells his no-fluoride-added Aztec Sea Salt to health food nutters like me, who flip out at the hint of any unnecessary adulteration of our food.

Other robust salts worth trying include Celtic Sea Salt. Like Aztec Sea Salt, it's harvested from the sea and allowed to dry in the sun, and is rich in trace minerals. Harvested on the coast of France, Celtic Sea Salt is slightly gray in color and has a bolder flavor than most other salts, making it a favorite of chefs around the world for its earthy, "old world" taste.

Himalayan salt, mined in Pakistan in the foothills of the Himalayas, has a pinkish color from its iron oxide content. Because it comes from ancient deposits, it is regarded by many as one of the purest salts on the market, which means fewer trace minerals but a clean taste.

## Bottom Line, Why the Confusion about Salt?

Why does this confusion about salt persist? Why so much back and forth in the research, which leaves us with more questions than answers about whether it's safe to eat? The problem isn't that the studies are necessarily wrong but that the entire structure of the salt argument is flawed.

Your genes might make you more sensitive to salt. In her bestselling book *The Body Ecology Diet,* Donna Gates explains that one of the main reasons some of our salt data is way off is that we fail to account for genetic sensitivity. "We literally need to do over all the studies," she says. She recommends eliminating study participants who are genetically sensitive to salt—namely, those who start to react negatively after about two tablespoons. "Let's see what happens," Donna suggests, "if they pull out all the people who are genetically salt sensitive and then use a high-quality, healthy salt" for the tests.

According to Donna, even if you're one of those salt-sensitive people, research shows you can still consume up to two teaspoons a day—about 4,600 mg of sodium. That's more than most people eating a healthy diet are consuming, so if you're not eating junk, you won't exceed your salt intake, even if you're salt sensitive.

The sweet spot for salt, like for most things, I've found, depends on a number of factors. But the bottom line is, it's hard to exceed healthy salt intake if you follow the three simple rules.

Bonus rule four? *Relax.* Which, as you'll find out next, is pretty much the only thing I can do for five days while I follow one of the weirdest but most effective health protocols I've ever experienced.

# CHAPTER 13

# NEED MORE ENERGY? DO NOTHING. WELL, KIND OF . . .

It's been four days since I've eaten anything. August 9, 2010, to be exact. No food. No tea. No juice. Nothing but completely pure, distilled water.

But don't worry, I'm not being held against my will at a terrorist camp in a country far away. I'm in Santa Rosa, California, the largest city in wine country, about an hour and a half north of San Francisco. Even more unusual is that I've actually asked to be here. Asked eagerly. In fact, I signed a waiver to prove it.

I'm voluntarily consuming nothing but water for five days. All in the name of health. Most people think this is crazy, and I have to admit, I did, too—at least until I met Alan Goldhamer.

Alan is a chiropractor and director of the True North Health Center, where he has supervised more than 10,000 water fasts since the clinic opened in 1984.

This is where I am now, experiencing firsthand a medically supervised water-only fast, structured from Alan's findings over three decades of clinical work. But even with all this experience, Alan is quick to deflect any credit for his success. He tells me that his mentor, Gerald Benesh, a chiropractor who co-founded the International Natural Hygiene Society, used to say that directing medically supervised water fasts was the best job in the world: "The body does all the healing and the patients do all the work, and all the doctor has to do is take credit for the good results."

"So," Alan says, "I thought, *Well, that's the job for me.*"

Alan's "nonwork" hasn't gone unnoticed. His clinic has been featured in *GQ* magazine and on *Nightline*. Both times, he says, they were probably looking to see just how quack-worthy water fasting was, but they came to the same conclusion: it works. Alan has published studies in peer-reviewed journals, giving water fasting more credibility in a still very traditional medical community. But most important for you and me, he may be stockpiling the most energy-boosting, detoxifying, and healing regimen on the planet.

It's not too far of a stretch to assume that you need to eat every day to be healthy. If you don't eat for a few months, you'll turn into worm food. But the truth is, most people won't die if they don't eat for a few days. In fact, Alan's premise is, they will get healthier.

The journey I'm on here is a shortcut to more energy and detoxification, but it's definitely not the only one. So if you think water fasting is too extreme, just remember "detoxification"—and I'll explain more as this little experiment unfolds.

## Rebooting Your Energy Hard Drive

When we pulled the RV into town a week earlier, I never thought that I, the guy who turns into a blood sugar–deprived monster when he doesn't eat every four to five hours, would be able to survive on just water. (The rule in our house is "Anything I say until I eat should be completely ignored.") But right now, 96 hours in, I feel fantastic. Probably better than I have in years. I glide when I walk. I feel sharp, quick, as if I could finish a crossword puzzle in record time or beat you at chess. Maybe it's an illusion, but whatever it is, I want more of it.

Alan tells me that what I'm doing is not complicated physiologically, by any means. Fasting is an age-old practice, done by humans for thousands of years. Jesus, Muhammad, and the Buddha all fasted. It's the oldest form of detox.

But what Alan does at True North is a little more thorough than just drinking water for 3, 5, 10, or 40 days. (Yes, 40.) What he does is called a controlled medical water fast. But even with that more com-plicated name, the process is actually quite basic. He uses a simple analogy: "By eliminating everything, which is what you do with fast-ing, it's like rebooting the hard drive in a computer. You shut the thing down, you turn it on, and it's amazing how much stuff just clears out."

I've wanted to experience a water fast firsthand ever since I heard Alan speak in April 2010. At first glance, it would be easy to assume he's an accountant or a financial planner. His hair is cut short and combed neatly. He dresses tidily, his button-down shirt always tucked in. He's not excessively nerdy, but I wouldn't put it past him to wear a pocket protector and defend his choice with statistics from some obscure study on the number of pocket-pen explosions over the last two decades.

While growing up in the Long Beach area of Southern California, Alan started learning about health and, more specifically, "natural hygiene." Natural hygiene refers to activating the body's restorative powers by allowing it to function in its purest state through regular fasting and a light vegetarian diet. With the aim of beating his child-hood friend in basketball, Alan would secretly read all he could about diet, including anything by Herbert Shelton and other notable natural hygienists of the time. It started to work—his game improved—but he couldn't resist tipping off his buddy to his research. They both adopted the same diet, almost immediately eliminating Alan's edge.

Alan's interest in diet and health lead him to Western State Chi-ropractic College in Portland, Oregon. From there, he went on to Pacific College of Osteopathic Medicine in Sydney, Australia, to study under hygienic physician Alex Burton, eventually doing an internship at Dr. Burton's Arcadia Health Centre, which specialized in medically supervised, water-only fasting. Upon his return to the United States in 1984, Alan and his wife, Jennifer Marano, also an osteopath, opened the True North Health Center. It's been going full tilt ever since.

At True North, Alan has used fasting to help people with all types of medical conditions of excess, from too much stress to overeating to consuming too much salt, oil, sugar, or coffee. These conditions didn't really apply to me when I signed up, since I was already a health pur-ist—though admittedly it wasn't working for me. But they applied to just about everyone else I knew, so I asked if I could film my five days of fasting to show on our video blog. I knew the topic would resonate with our viewers. Alan agreed.

But it wasn't just for our viewers, of course. I was secretly hoping that maybe this treatment (or nontreatment, if you want to call it that) would help with my low energy and the acne on my face and back that was still unresolved from my previous raw food experiment, even though I'd stopped my vegan diet a few months earlier. Since water fasting is a process in which by not eating you let the body naturally bring itself back into balance, I thought maybe it would help with the adrenal and hormonal wreckage from my extreme diet.

Four days in—and way past the initial *Am I really not going to eat for five days?* anxiety—it's definitely working. I feel energy radiating out of my body. I'm quickly becoming an evangelist and feel the need to tell everyone, ill or not, about water fasting. By healing people with serious illnesses, Alan has found a secret to maximizing the body's potential energy.

## Miracle Results, but No One's Heard of Them

Alan's healing crusade really started gaining steam with his work on patients with high blood pressure. He focused his attention there because it was low-hanging fruit. "High blood pressure is the leading contributing cause of death and disability in industrialized countries," Alan says. "The majority of people, by the time they reach 65, if they aren't dead from something else, have high blood pressure." The consequences, of course, can be devastating—heart failure and stroke. But high blood pressure is easy to measure reliably, Alan explains, and is responsive to treatment. "Virtually everybody who comes in with hypertension normalizes," he tells me.

In fact, they do better than on drugs. Alan doesn't mince words: "Medical management of high blood pressure sucks." Medication fails to deal with the underlying causes. So he and his team enlisted Cornell researcher T. Colin Campbell to run a cohort study. They gathered 174 patients, had them do medically supervised water fasts, and tracked them for 12 years.[1] The result was that all 174 people in the study lowered their blood pressure enough to eliminate the need for medication. The water fast reduced blood pressure an average of 60 points more than the accepted medical treatment being used around the world. In my view, Alan should be hailed as a hero. But while every medical doctor knows the name of the most effective beta-blocker, diuretic, or calcium-channel blocker—common drugs for hypertension—few have ever heard of Alan Goldhamer, DC.

But they will soon. Because Alan didn't stop at hypertension. He noticed that his patients with high blood pressure were also seeing improvements in other conditions. His medical testing proved it. Water fasting was making them better.

At that point, Alan widened his focus. If a patient had a condition that could be loosely related to diseases of excess like high blood pressure, blood-sugar imbalance, arthritis, leaky gut, obesity, allergies, or stress, he would recommend giving fasting a try—with a caveat. He told patients he had no idea how their body would react, or if fasting would work for them. The best he could promise was a clean room to sleep in, two daily medical check-ins, and all the water they could drink.

It sounds unbelievable, but this why I came to True North—to see if it was true. Now, after months of feeling physically sluggish and emotionally drained from trying so many methods that didn't work, I feel fantastic. Doing nothing is proving to be better than all the supplement protocols, diet regimens, and electronic medical devices I've tried. I can get out of bed early. I can move better. I have energy throughout the day. I didn't know how low my energy really was until I found out how good I could feel.

And that's one of the biggest problems we all face with health and fitness. We don't know how bad we feel until we feel good. You don't have to do a five-day water fast to restore your energy. You just have to take the basic principles of water fasting and use them to your advantage.

## Stop the Energy-Suck Cycle

It's Day 1 of my fast. I walk into Michael Klapper's office on the second floor of the True North Health Center. Michael is a traditionally trained medical doctor from the University of Illinois who used to practice urgent care and anesthesiology. Now you could say he's gone rogue. He's vegan. He eats almost no salt, oil, or sugar. Tall, thin, and gray haired, he looks better than most doctors in their 50s, let alone late 60s, which he is.

Michael has totally bought into the idea of fasting. "If there was a pill that did what 21 days on water will do for you, we would all be rich," he says. "It's a powerful therapeutic modality. Blood pressures come down, blood sugars even out, and joints cool off."

As we run through my intake questionnaire, I explain that I'm here mainly as research but also to see if water fasting does anything for my adrenal health, acne, and energy levels. Clearly influenced by Alan's *We just remove everything to see what happens* mantra, Michael says I might be surprised by what happens during and after the five days of my fast.

He asks me about my daily food habits and is happy that I don't drink coffee or eat sugar regularly. Relying on them for energy can make you a real-life zombie, he notes. My conclusions about sugar and caffeine, as outlined in previous chapters, apply to a body that is running smoothly. When you have low energy, however, it means your body is like an out-of-tune guitar. The fix is to bring it back to the right pitch.

To do this, you have to remove the factors that are making you sluggish, as well as those that are giving you a false sense of energy. Yuri Elkaim, author of *The All Day Energy Diet,* calls caffeine and sugar "energy impostors." If you've been relying on them to pick you up or keep you going throughout the day, your body has started to chemically depend on them as an energy source.

The adrenal glands, which sit on top of the kidneys, play an important role in assisting the pancreas with blood sugar regulation. Too much sugar in your diet and blood interferes with your body's ability to stay in balance and overworks both the pancreas and the adrenals as they try to keep your blood sugar in check. The more overworked your adrenals, the lower your energy. Then, as your energy wanes, you look for energy from other sources—usually more sugar and caffeine.

Caffeine and the adrenals work together—or against each other—in another way. Caffeine stimulates the adrenals to produce more of the hormones epinephrine and norepinephrine (also known as adrenaline and noradrenaline), which jack up your heart rate and raise your blood sugar, providing an energy jolt. Using caffeine to stimulate your body's own energy production works in the short term but is devastating in the long term. The more caffeine you take in, the more overstimulated your adrenal glands, and eventually they cut production.

Not only is adrenal health related to energy, but it's also related to longevity. In traditional Chinese medicine, the kidneys and adrenal glands are the most important organs in the body for health and long life. Taoist practitioners devote a great deal of time to practices that conserve subtle energy originating from the kidney and adrenal complex. Taoists believe that we are born with a certain amount of energy that is enough to last our lifetime, as long as we live a balanced and harmonious life.

My consult done, I thank Dr. Klapper and start packing up my camera and sound equipment. I find myself thinking about my adrenals—the two little globs of gooey flesh sitting atop my kidneys that guard my energy with the best of intentions but can easily be distracted by a hit of sugar or caffeine. Those poor addicts. We enable them all the time. The only way to get them straight is to temporarily cut off their supply, which is one reason a water fast works: you're prohibited from eating sugar, drinking caffeine, or taking any other stimulant.

The good news is, you don't need to do a water fast to go cold turkey. To detox from these energy vampires, you just need to be in a place where you can't access sugar, caffeine, and stimulants long enough for your adrenals and pancreas to take a break and your body to reset. So, energy and detox solution numero uno is to do a sugar and caffeine fast, removing them both from your diet for at least two weeks. You won't die, I promise.

Physician Mark Hyman paints a rosy picture of this type of detox diet. "When you shut off the hormones and the brain chemistry that are driving these cravings," he says, "change happens very quickly. Within a day or so, you literally are eating and doing a few simple lifestyle practices in a way that quickly resets your whole system."

If the idea of stopping cold sounds daunting, there are some substitutes you can put on your shopping list to help you make it through your fast. To curb sugar cravings, add more protein to your diet, such as nuts, eggs, protein shakes, or grass-fed meat. Many people even swear by a splash of apple cider vinegar in a glass of water to satisfy a sweet tooth.

Giving your system a break from sugar and caffeine is just one aspect of balancing your energy, however. To get the whole picture, you need to go deeper, and I mean that literally. You have to go down your throat, through your stomach, into your small intestine. That kind of deep.

## Give Your Belly a Break

The accommodations at True North are surprisingly nice. Annmarie and I have been to all different types of health retreat centers, from rustic cabins in Costa Rica to simple adobe units in the southern Arizona high desert to the luxurious condos at We Care Detox Spa and Spiritual Retreat in Palm Desert, California, but the units here are perfect for doing what you do on a water fast—lounge around.

Right now it's summer, so it's 90 degrees or so in the daytime, then drops into the 60s at night. It's Day 2 of my fast. Inside the room it's warm, so the door is open and the lights are off. There's enough sun coming through the open blinds to make it bright enough to see where I'm going when I move around, which is infrequently.

It would be a perfect day to sit on the lounge chairs out in the courtyard, but I'm having a mini-crisis. I'm hungry, of course. I haven't eaten in 36 hours. But I'm also obsessing about something more personal: I haven't pooped since I got here. I'm usually one-or-two-times-a-day regular. But right now, I'm constipated.

Since I have nothing else to do besides drink about six more glasses of water today, I do a little research on what might be happening. Essentially, my entire evac system has taken a break. This is actually a good thing, it seems. While my intestines are healing during the fasting process, they're also rebuilding the mucosal lining that runs all the way down my digestive tract to my personal emergency exit. Since most of us are eating way too much food and way too many foods that cause gut irritation and inflammation, it's a good idea to give the digestive system a rest. If you have gut inflammation and continue to eat foods that inflame it, you're not going to heal.

So what does gut inflammation mean to your health? More than you may think. It's linked to allergies, skin disorders, arthritis, diarrhea, chronic illness, and poor immune function. It's also linked to fatigue, which is most relevant for this chapter on energy. You're not at your personal energy pinnacle if your gut is inflamed.

Alan explains to me what's at work here: something called *gut leakage.* When your intestinal mucosa, the lining of the digestive tract, is inflamed, "it absorbs proteins from the gut that really shouldn't be in the bloodstream," he says. "And in genetically vulnerable people, that appears to trigger immunological responses. Sometimes the body will begin reacting to its own tissues. If it happens to react to your colon tissues, it might manifest as symptoms of colitis. If it's in the joints, we might call it arthritis. If it's in the lungs, you've got asthma and related conditions like psoriasis and eczema."

With all these conditions, in which the immune system has become confused and is turning on its own tissues, fasting can be helpful, Alan says. "Number one, you're not eating anything, so there are no dietary antigens to stimulate the system. Number two, the cascade of healing issues that happens in fasting facilitates the resolution of gut leakage." Result? "The inflammation comes down."

So when you stop eating food or, for the less adventurous, eliminate the foods that commonly cause gut inflammation, your gut will start to heal. This, in turn, will likely help with anything else inflammation-related you may be experiencing, including reduced energy levels.

As I sit here on this La-Z-Boy, feeling calm, my gut is healing. This makes not eating food for three and a half more days seem worth it. I take a sip of water. It tastes strangely dry. Like a water sommelier, I'm starting to appreciate the different textures and flavors of water. This one has notes of nothingness, with a little bit of crisp at the mid-palate and quite a bit of sticky tongue on the finish.

Energy and detox principle number two: gut healing. Check.

## HEALING THE GUT WITHOUT WATER FASTING

The truth is, water fasting isn't for everyone. If you can't see yourself subsisting on water alone for even 24 hours but you want to repair your gut, hope is not lost. Here are some alternative ways:

**Do a three-day cleanse.** On our website, we outline one called the Weekend Detox at www.RenegadeHealth.com/weekendcleanse. It's perfect for first timers and people who don't have the time or inclination to lie around for five or more days.

**Do a juice fast.** For three to five days, drink only freshly made vegetable juices. Juicing extracts the water and nutrients from the veggies, so you absorb a lot of nutrients without having to digest the fiber. Kris Carr, author of *Crazy Sexy Wellness,* has juice recipes on her website, http://kriscarr.com/recipes/juices-smoothies/.

**Do a smoothie fast.** The smoothie fast is the same as the juice fast, but instead of juices you drink green smoothies for three to five days, at breakfast, lunch, dinner, and in between. With smoothies you're getting the entire veggie, pulp and all. Even though blending breaks down the fiber, there's still some digestion involved. On the plus side, the slower release of nutrients prevents blood sugar spikes.

**Regularly take probiotics.** Your gut maintains an ecosystem of gut flora that allow you to properly digest foods and extract the nutrients you need from them. The trouble begins when this balance is upset. To restore your microflora to optimal balance, take probiotics—dietary supplements containing "friendly" gut bacteria.

**Start taking digestive enzymes.** Protein supplements that help the gut break down food, digestive enzymes are another way to repair the gut and increase your energy.

### I'm Failing the Last One

It's Day 4—one and a half more days of not eating to go. I have to admit that physically this has been much easier than I thought it would be. I'm weak, but I don't have any aches or pains or severe lightheadedness. My teeth are covered in a sticky film I can feel when I run my tongue over them, but otherwise, no complaints.

Emotionally, however, I'm losing it. I have no idea what to do when I don't have anything to do. I wonder if being comfortable with stillness might be one of my lifetime challenges to master. I've never been able to sit for anything, anywhere. I can't do yoga. I can't meditate. I'm a pacer. Being here, confined at the center, is maddening. I've already read two books, so now I'm fishing for ideas and impatiently waiting for tomorrow so I can fill up an hour with filming and editing another video.

Shea, the friend who's joined us for a fast of her own, says that her boyfriend could bring in a DVD or two to help pass the time. I'm not usually a TV guy, but the thought of being able to burn two hours and get closer to the end of my fast is exciting. She calls him, and a few hours later, we're watching the first episode of *Breaking Bad*, a drama series about a chemistry teacher who turns into a methamphetamine kingpin. Only a few minutes in, my boredom fades. We watch five episodes in a row.

Day 5 is more *Breaking Bad*. Aside from filming a daily video, it's essentially the only thing we do. But if I had known that *Breaking Bad* was such a deep, involved, and dark story before I got hooked, I think I would have opted instead for a few seasons of *Friends* or *Seinfeld* during my fast. *Breaking Bad* keeps us all at a constant level of anxiety, waiting for what will happen next. A good TV drama does this well, but I know what stress like this does to my body.

In truth, I'm not fully fasting, at least at an emotional level. When I think of pure emotional fasting, I think of Buddhism, and right now, I can't imagine a monk on retreat in a temple in Asia sneaking away to check out where Walter White and Jesse Pinkman are cooking meth.

For most of us, when we're not holed up in a condo in Santa Rosa, experiencing stress in overabundance is just a part of every day. What's sad is that we accept the emotional roller coaster of modern life as normal. That bout of road rage you almost had on the way to work this morning? Normal. That anxiety about your finances that hangs around like a hungry wolf at the door? Par for the course. Quiet desperation over the to-do list that leaves little time for rest and rejuvenation? Business as usual. As we contend every day with so-called normal life, our adrenals are constantly firing, gradually lowering our immune response and making us susceptible to everything from the flu to flat-out exhaustion. We burn out.

For some people, the way out is to leave everything behind and retreat to a monastery in Thailand. For the rest of us, the key is finding a way to consistently address our ballooning stress. I've mentioned tapping, but there are a variety of other practices you can do. Many people swear by journaling, as it gives them an empty page on which to dump all their troublesome emotions, while others are devoted practitioners of tai chi or yoga, gently working out their feelings through their bodies. Maybe all you need to de-stress is to go for a long walk and get away from everybody. Whatever you choose, gaining some freedom from your emotions is paramount.

For me, emotional calm is by far the hardest of the three fasting principles to master. I'm resigned to a lifelong practice of managing, not conquering, stress.

But we have an entire evening and season two to go. Despite all my talk about lessening anxiety and adrenal stress, the show is just too good to stop watching. Might as well binge now and manage later. So tonight consists of more *Breaking Bad,* a half-dozen glasses of water, and lots of lying on the couch.

## NUTRIENTS FOR ENERGY

Nutrients are essential for keeping your energy up. Here are a few key ones you don't want to run low on:

**Magnesium.** This mineral is a key component of ATP, the fuel source for every cell in your body. You can boost your magnesium levels through supplementation and through dark leafy greens, cereals, and nuts.

**Iron.** Hemoglobin in red blood cells ferries oxygen to all your tissues and organs. Iron is a major component of hemoglobin. There are high levels of iron in red meat, but if you're looking to cut back you can also get iron from dark leafy greens, beans, and broccoli.

**Folate.** A member of the B vitamin family, folate, or vitamin B9, plays an important role in maintaining your DNA. It's readily available in many types of legumes (black-eyed peas, lentils, and pinto beans) as well as in asparagus, broccoli, and spinach.

## All Done

A plate of mango, papaya, watermelon, and figs sits in front of me. I pick up a piece of mango with my fork and let it touch my tongue. The flavor is intense. Kind of orgasmic—at least by mouth standards. I want it to last forever, so I chew every piece 40 times or more.

The last five days have changed me. So much so that I actually had anxiety about eating again. *What if I started eating and lost this constant buzz that I feel?* The buzz is addicting.

Everything seems as if it's been reset. My eyes are clear. My breath doesn't smell. My mind is sharp. I'm not gassy or bloated. My digestion and evac system are working super-smoothly. Even my sleep is perfect, retuned to my natural circadian rhythms. Over the last five days, I've eliminated any stimulating food or drink and allowed my gut to heal. I've also identified a source of low energy that I'll address, and I've taken—or should have taken—an emotional break. So, three out of four.

Regardless, I still have more energy than I have in years. I hope it won't go away soon. I know that energy is a slippery thing to contain. It slides away when you're not looking and doesn't come back until you have to sacrifice for it.

You don't have to sacrifice as much as I did—not eating for five days—to kick-start your energy levels, though for some of you, a water fast will be the most effective way. What's more important for your own detoxification is to think like someone who's fasting and use the three basic principles: reset your body from excessive stimulants, heal your gut, and calm your emotions. When you do that, you, too, are likely to feel as if you're radiating bolts of energy.

Alan assures me that my body has done some deep cleansing and that the way I feel won't disappear the minute I leave. He's right. A few days later I still feel like an electric generator. I've had a complete reboot.

## Real-Time Check-in: July 2014

It's been four years since the water fast. I haven't done one since, but I've tried to live with the three fasting principles in mind. I've particularly focused on them on this most recent journey.

Having removed coffee and 95 percent of the sugar I was eating, I'm following a plant-strong diet, eliminating most dairy, wheat, grains, soy, and eggs, but including some animal foods, as if I were living in a Blue Zone. I've cut out 95 percent of the foods that can cause gut irritation. I've also done a few three-day cleanses, including our Weekend Cleanse program, to rest my body and restore my energy. I have to admit, though, that I watched the entire *Breaking Bad* series again in March. That's energy-depleting binge behavior I still need to address.

Regardless of my resistance to emotional fasting, the overall results of the water fast are positive. I'm running regularly and getting faster. I'm at my lowest weight since January, down to 191 pounds from 223. My skin and eyes look better. I don't ask Annmarie if I look fat three times a day.

Above all, my mind is really clear. During my anything-organic binge, I wasn't as concerned about low energy as about my brain. It was starting to do some pretty strange things. Sometimes, I'd forget what I was saying in mid-sentence. Other times, I couldn't recall a name or detail that normally I would know. It was almost as if my brain wasn't firing properly—like a car that wouldn't start on a cold day.

So, before I fix the wiring of my own personal command center, I have to tell you why it's so important to do so in the first place. Fittingly, the last part of the story starts where it all began—Pittsburgh. This time, however, the situation is much different from getting an RV stuck on a country road. My grandfather is dying.

# CHAPTER 14

# MY ENTENMANN'S-CAKE-EATING GRANDFATHER SHOWS ME THE LAST SECRET OF THE LONGEST-LIVED PEOPLE

I'm at a Starbucks about ten minutes from the airport, drinking a green tea and writing a bit before I have to pick up my mother, whose flight lands at 12:30 P.M. She and I have come to join my aunt, who lives here, to visit my grandfather, who's under hospice care.

I'm doing all right considering how emotional I was while booking my plane ticket two days ago. This may be because I haven't seen my grandfather yet. I keep picturing him as he was throughout my childhood: broad shouldered, with arms strong enough to toss my brother and me high in the air as we play in his backyard pool. His features are sharp and masculine, his beard neatly trimmed but thick. For this visit, though, my mother has warned me that his body has started to break down. He's weak. It's possible he may not even want us to see him like this—his pride is not as frail as his 95-year-old body.

It's difficult for me to imagine him dying in bed with us sitting around him. But there's a very real possibility that this is how the next three days will play out. I've never seen anyone die, and I'm certain I don't ever need to in order to feel complete. But instead of spending any more time ruminating, I force myself to think about what a feat it is that my grandfather has lived for nearly a century.

Just about everything I've done in the name of health is to figure out how to live longer. Yet until recently, I've always overlooked the fact that my very own grandfather is a living example of longevity. I've looked at long-lived cultures and scientific studies for clues, but my grandfather is likely as close as I'll get to 95, unless I get there myself.

And while it's evident that he's dying now, 50 days ago you wouldn't have known. You would have found him out on his tractor, mowing his lawn; or watching the news on TV; or trying to contact his local councilman to complain about his well water, which was contaminated by fracking nearby. He was still as sharp, as capable, and as stubborn as always. If this is how I'll be living just before I die, I'll be satisfied.

But my mind bends every time I think about Pop-Pop and his advanced age. Over the last two years, I've done my best to pry into his daily habits, but I still have only a few clues as to why he lived so long and my other three grandparents did not. In fact, there was far more about Pop-Pop that pointed to an early death, but for whatever reason, he endured.

Born Albert Molino, my grandfather never followed any health guru, diet, or exercise regimen. In fact, from a health perspective, he did many things I would strongly advise against. He was a soldier in World War II and saw his friends die in Germany. He lived in Pittsburgh, where the smoke from the steel mills was so thick it darkened his first 37 years—and his lungs. He owned a car service shop for decades, inhaling on a daily basis noxious oils, fumes, and chemicals, many of which are now banned. He smoked for more than half of his life. He is painfully stubborn. For the last 15 or so years he has done all his food shopping at Walmart and the Entenmann's Bakery outlet. Based on the odds that science would give him, he shouldn't have lived this long. For that matter, the odds that his personal development gave him were also poor. After my grandmother died 18 years ago, he wanted to die as well. So I can't even attribute his longevity to a positive mental attitude—at least not for the past 18 years. But he's never been on a regular medication, let alone the two or more prescription drugs that most Americans are taking by age 60.[1] And he continued to work in his yard, mowing the lawn and gardening, and to tinker in his basement tool shop until he had a small stroke in early March—just six weeks before I went to see him.

Clearly, Pop-Pop has not lived the pure, no-gluten, spirulina-munching, chemical-free life my favorite health gurus have, so what is the secret of his longevity?

## A Clue

I'm sure it's complicated and simple all at once. Of course, some part of his longevity can be attributed to his genes. But the challenge with chalking longevity up to good genes is that there are people with good genes who die young. Even people with almost identical genomes don't live as long as each other. According to the Laboratory of Survival and Longevity at the Max Planck Institute for Demographic Research in Germany, identical twins die, on average, ten years apart.[2]

Another part of Pop-Pop's longevity is probably luck. To my knowledge he was never exposed to any major diseases or rare infections that weakened his immune system, even as he grew older. (I don't know this for sure, but he's never really been sick.) It could be that he ate straight from the family garden as a kid. It's certainly not because he took supplements—he never did. But apart from these possible variables, there's one that I know for sure contributed to his longevity—that maybe even was the foundation of it. It was revealed to me about four years ago on a visit.

Pop-Pop calls me into his office. It's a small room in his home, 30 miles northeast of Pittsburgh. The town, if you can even call it that, is a small community named Apollo. My grandfather's house is on a country road that has about a 50 percent chance of being indexed by Google Maps. He's lived here for 20 or more years, ever since the state bought his previous home to build a turnpike extension. In his office, he has a computer desktop setup that rivals a hotshot programmer's: two monitors, a printer, a webcam, and a slide scanner—all this to take the slides of my grandmother's artwork and archive them in digital files. This is the project he took on after he couldn't tinker in his basement machine shop any more. He worked almost into his

90s building chemical mixers that were sold to labs. But now he has adapted. He's the only nonagenarian I know who is regularly firing off emails, scanning images, burning CDs, and posting comments on all relevant Hillary Clinton message boards.

Pop-Pop wants to show me some of the art he has scanned and says he needs some help setting up Skype to connect with his camera. As I start to connect the webcam, I notice an embossed label stuck to the top of his monitor. On it is a phrase:

*When you lose the mental game, you lose the physical one.*

I point to it. He just nods his head. His reaction indicates that this is not something he thinks should surprise me. His brain is simply wired to think this way and believe it's true. I wonder if this is one of the main reasons he's still here, regardless of his diet, genetics, or exercise habits. What he thinks on an everyday basis is likely a significant contributing factor to his long life.

## Mastering the Mental Game

Now, in Starbucks, I've convinced myself that my grandfather's philosophy of life is one of the main reasons he's still here. I'm wondering if I have the same belief system. And if so, will I live as long as he? Then I get a text from my mother: *Landed . . . checked baggage . . . will call when I get bag.* I'll have to reflect more on this later.

Proving the extent to which someone's thinking plays a role in his longevity is not an easy task. With so many variables, it's hard to assign all the credit to just one. That would be like saying the ingredient chocolate *is* the brownie. Yes, chocolate definitely makes it a brownie, but you don't have a brownie without all the other ingredients, too. It's the same with longevity. You can't single out exercise and ignore someone's sleep habits, diet, friendships, interests, and emotional well-being. I'm attempting to prove that how you use your brain is a variable that cannot be left out. While to some it may sound like a woo-woo, feel-good theory, it's not. There is already science behind it.

As part of a wide-ranging study of cognitive function and aging in the United Kingdom, researchers tracked 12,470 senior citizens over

16 years. They wanted to see if mental cognition—*thought agility,* as I call it—correlates with a longer life span. The results were positive for thinkers. The researchers found that on average, a 65-year-old man from the lowest social bracket, with the lowest education, occupation, and social engagement, could expect to live to age 68, with cognitive impairment for the last 4.3 of those years. At the other end of the spectrum, an educated 65-year-old man at the top of the social scale could expect to live to almost 81, with dementia for only the last 1.6 years.[3]

The famous Nun Study is an ongoing longitudinal study on aging and Alzheimer's disease. It began in 1986, when epidemiologist David Snowdon started examining the lives of 678 elderly sisters at a convent in Missouri, in the hope of gaining insight into the origins of Alzheimer's. Reading journal entries written by the sisters when they were in their 20s, Snowdon noticed that those who gave the most detailed accounts, displaying what Snowdon termed "idea density," were less likely to develop Alzheimer's or other dementia as they aged. What's more, the sisters who had written the most complex entries ended up living longer.[4]

These are just two examples, but they show that an active brain contributes to longer life. Clearly, longevity studies based only on factors like diet and exercise are shortsighted.

## At Death's Door?

My grandfather is sleeping when we walk into his room at the assisted living facility. He's just returned from the hospital. The doctors released him back here for hospice care. He could die in an hour or a day or a week. We don't know. His eyes are a quarter open, and his breathing is labored. My mother, my aunt, and I gather around him, openly shedding tears, waiting for his last breath. We put on a CD of "Lara's Theme" from *Dr. Zhivago*—his and my grandmother's favorite.

"Ooohahhhahgh." My mother, my aunt, and I look at each other. He's speaking.

We lean in, thinking these are his last words. I'm frustrated because I can't hear them. I want to take them with me, but there's no making out what he's saying. I turn down the music to see if I can hear better.

But after a few minutes of this, he starts to sound clearer, forming words we can understand. It turns out this isn't his last hurrah just yet. The morphine they gave him at the hospital is wearing off. He begins to tell us that we need a plan.

"A plan?" my mother asks.

"Nothing is worth it if you don't have a plan," he slurs.

His plan, just as any half-libertarian, half-Democrat, fuzzy-on-opiates 95-year-old would have it, is to buy a bunch of land and live off the grid in a community—all the family together. We all have skills that could keep us alive and healthy, he says. We could escape the corrupt government. We could live together and enjoy the rest of our time here. "We don't need much money; we'll all be together," he says.

As I listen, my mother and aunt agree with him, even though we all know this will never happen. What else can they do? Deny a dying man a wish? So we play along with the fantasy for a while. As we do, I start thinking again about Pop-Pop's longevity. I look at the desk on the other side of the room and see his computer monitor. On the top is the same embossed label. He's never given up on this mantra: *When you lose the mental game, you lose the physical one.* Even now, his mind is still working. He's still making plans. Moving forward. Against all odds, he has a dream and is still fighting for it to come true.

As I'm running this through my head, he stops speaking in mid-sentence. We all notice and quickly look to his chest to see if he's still breathing. He is. He then points to the nurse standing halfway between the doorway and the bed, not wanting to interrupt us. As she starts talking to my mother and aunt, he turns his head slowly, touches my hand with his, and winks. It could be because he thinks she's cute, but I doubt it. The look and the wink are to indicate that this plan is our family secret. No outsiders allowed.

My Pop-Pop didn't die during the three days I was in Pittsburgh. In fact, he got stronger. The final two days I was there, he became more and more coherent—and, of course, more stubborn. He ripped out his catheter because he wanted get up and go to the bathroom himself, and he grumbled about the lousy food. Before I left, I held his hand as I sat on the side of his bed. I knew it was the last time I'd see him, but there was still a part of me that believed he was going to live for another ten years. With a mind like his—always working, planning, thinking, learning—anything was possible. I wondered if my mind would keep me around for as long as his had served him. Then he kicked me out in the nicest of ways. "Go back to your family. You don't need to be here with this old man. Go make memories," he said.

On the flight back to Oakland, I send an email to a friend of mine, Jim Kwik. Jim is a memory and speed-reading trainer, and I ask him for a reintroduction to psychiatrist Daniel Amen. Daniel is one of the most sought-after holistic brain specialists in the United States, probably in the world. At his clinics, he scans, diagnoses, and heals the brains of people of all ages, with all sorts of cognitive disorders. Daniel's scan identifies how much of the brain is working and how much isn't. His most recent focus—studying and improving the brain functioning of ex-NFL football players who have sustained brain trauma throughout their careers—has pushed his work into the mainstream. A few years back, he invited me to come to his facility and get a brain scan, so I could see what my gray matter looks like under the hood. At that time, we were traveling in the RV, and the invite slipped through the cracks.

My grandfather never had a chance to have his brain looked at objectively, but modern science has evolved to make this possible. Which is bittersweet for me. I would almost rather not know what my brain looks like. What if it's totally wrecked? I played football in high school, which gives me a higher probability of having a damaged brain. I wasn't an angel, either. I did drugs in college. I drank heavily. Smoked. What would a scan that shows I really messed up my brain do to my thoughts about longevity? Would I give up, thinking there's no hope? I feared my brain wouldn't look as good as my grandfather's, which right up to the end was still functioning better than some brains 50 years younger than his.

If my theory on brain health is correct—that a healthy, happy, always-learning brain is a secret to longevity—it's in my absolute best interest to get the scan. And with the results, to make it my mission to have the healthiest brain on the planet. My grandfather is right: I need to be with my family and make memories for as long as I physically can. (Then you can take me out back and shoot me.) I'll just have to overcome all odds, think like my grandfather, and make a plan.

A day later, Daniel Amen writes back. It's a go.

## Not Smarter Than a Monkey

Thirty-six days later, I'm sitting in a dark room alone at the Amen Clinic in Brisbane, California, 15 minutes south of San Francisco, on the Bay. I'm staring at a black computer screen that is flashing white letters at varying speeds. I've been instructed to hit the spacebar for every letter except X.

*J, spacebar. L, spacebar. G, spacebar. R, spacebar. R, spacebar. X, spacebar . . .*

"Fuck!" I say out loud. I'm maybe three minutes in, and I can't tell my Xs from any other letter. As the lab tech injected an isotope solution through the IV in my arm, he told me I would be doing this exercise for 14 minutes. I wonder if my inability to be perfect at this test is evidence that my brain is a swampy mess. I have a good run for a few minutes, but then my mind wanders again, and I hit the spacebar after another X. *A monkey could do better than this,* I think.

When the 14 minutes is up, the tech takes me into a large, cold, tiled room. There are two scanning machines here. Essentially, the scan will register all the places the isotope has gone since that computer made me feel like an inferior human.

"Just 20 minutes, and I'll be back," the tech says.

Next thing I know he's standing over me. The scan is done. I had fallen asleep. I groggily ask him if I can stay there longer and nap. He laughs, but I'm serious. My brain and body are tired.

## Unlocking Your Superhero Brain

The first time I meet Jim Kwik is in his office in White Plains, New York. I'm there with a group of ten people to take his half-day course on how to read faster. With a name like Kwik (pronounced "Quick"), it's ironic—and fitting—that he's in the field of brain processing speed enhancement. But the brain-training table wasn't always set for Jim.

At age five, he suffered a brain injury when he fell headfirst into an iron radiator and was knocked unconscious. He has no recollection of the event, but its effect on him was evident. "I was slow to learn," Jim says. "I was not only a slow reader, I was also slow to learn how to read and understand things. This had its physiological effects as well. I was shy because of it. I would actually make myself sick when I had to give any kind of book report. I would literally induce anxiety that made me sick so I could get out of doing work in school." Jim eventually learned to read by reading comic books that his parents and aunt and uncle bought for him. "I would stay up late reading those comic books," he recalls. "It was the only way I could learn."

You wouldn't think that someone who, as a child, had a brain injury and read nothing but comic books would later become a world-class brain trainer, but Jim has. He's done lectures and training at Harvard and New York University, and for corporate clients like Fox, Virgin, Nike, and Zappos. His private clients include A-list celebrities, global business leaders, and royalty. Jim's story took a turn when he realized that his brain learned differently from the brains of his classmates.

"In school they taught you *what* to learn but not *how* to learn," he says. So he started studying everything about his brain. His self-esteem improved overnight as he realized the potential locked away in those 100 billion brain cells. "But I still couldn't reconcile why we forget things or don't remember where we put our car keys," he says. "So I started to study adult learning theory and neuroscience and multiple intelligence. Anything I could get my hands on to figure out how the brain worked. About a month into it, a light switch went on."

Jim had discovered how to access parts of his brain he'd never been able to activate before. And with practice, he started to understand in a way he never had. His focus became clear. He could finally concentrate. He was able to remember more than he thought possible. His transformation was so astounding that he started teaching others what he'd learned. What if there was another kid out there who had the same problems he'd experienced at school? What if some of his classmates were having their potential held back in the classroom?

Jim's story is inspiring. You *can* change your brain. But he also sees the challenges we face as technology digs deeper into our everyday lives. Technology can actually change the chemistry of your body, triggering the release of neurotransmitters, especially dopamine, known as the brain's "reward chemical." If you spend more time on Facebook or Pinterest than you do talking to human beings, this is happening to you. Jim explains, "Every time you see that somebody likes or shares your posts, your body reacts chemically. Every time you get one of those notifications on your phone, you get your dopamine fix. You wonder why people are getting these technology addictions, but it's clear when you understand that they're getting their serotonin fix, they're getting their oxytocin. An emotional cocktail is flushed into our nervous system that always keeps us on."

Dopamine, serotonin, and oxytocin are feel-good chemicals that many of us are actually underproducing, so why would boosting them be bad? For one thing, they aren't meant to be "on" all the time. These neurotransmitters are supposed to do their job and then turn off. In excess, they can actually harm us. Even serotonin, which normally induces calm, at high doses causes jitters, nausea, even hallucinations. Pursuit of the never-ending hit keeps us out of brain states that are essential to learning, creativity, and physical and emotional well-being.

There are four different brain states, categorized by brain wave frequencies: alpha, beta, theta, and delta. Since we're constantly bombarded by technology, we spend most of our time in beta—the most awake state—or delta, the brain wave of sleep. "We're not spending as much time in the alpha or theta state," Jim says, "and these are the nourishing states for the brain. These are the states we go into when we rejuvenate and replenish. Research suggests that some learning challenges, especially with kids and attention deficit, arise from not spending any time in these middle states."

Alpha is the best state for learning. Meditating, doing visualization exercises, practicing conscious breathing, and listening to music with nature sounds or to baroque classical music at 60 beats a minute are effective means of lowering brain activity from the hyper-alert beta state to alpha.

All this is instructive, but it still doesn't explain why my grandfather is still around after nine-and-a-half decades. I tell Jim about Pop-Pop and the quote on his computer, thinking he'll point me toward some science on the subject. Instead, he shares a personal story.

"My grandmother died last year at 97, and she was old chronologically but she was young mentally." I think of Pop-Pop as Jim describes his grandmother reading the newspaper, watching the news on CNN, watching *Jeopardy*, doing crossword puzzles, playing mahjong—a traditional Chinese strategy game—and monitoring her investments. "The whole thing comes down to the concept of 'Use it or lose it,'" Jim adds. "Your brain is like a muscle: it grows stronger with use."

## TIPS FOR A HEALTHY BRAIN

Like a muscle, the brain goes stronger with use, says learning expert Jim Kwik. To keep your brain fit, he suggests:

**Move your body.** "As your body moves, your brain grooves," Jim says. You make better connections in your brain. Exercise is an obvious solution for brain health, and for a lot of people, standing or moving around while they're learning new information helps them retain it better. If you're one of those people, try a treadmill desk.

**Seek out novelty.** The brain thrives on new things. Dedicate yourself to lifelong learning, to mastering new skills, Jim suggests. "It's up to you what new things you explore. It can be a movement, a dance, a musical instrument, a subject, a foreign language. All of that is good for your brain."

**Draw up a not-to-do list.** The most productive people, Jim says, "have things they just will not do or will not take on because they understand their productivity is about maximizing their amount of output per input." Topping your not-to-do list should be things that distract you from your primary goals. "Your brain mostly is a deletion creature and is actually looking for things to just ignore and stop focusing on," Jim says. What a relief.

**Do a brain dump.** Another way to decrease the load on your brain is to put things down on paper. "Many people don't have focus because they have multiple 'windows' open, just like they would on the computer," Jim says. "Even if the windows are minimized, they're still taking up space and processing power." To free up your mind, Jim suggests jotting down ideas on a whiteboard. I recently painted part of a wall in my office with chalkboard paint for making notes.

**Do brain exercises.** There are a variety of exercises aimed at keeping your brain active and alert, such as the "neurobics" in Lawrence Katz's book *Keep Your Brain Alive*. Katz, a neurobiologist at Duke University Medical Center, suggests simple brain-body activities like eating or brushing your teeth with your nondominant hand, playing table tennis, or changing the radio station you listen to—even just wriggling your toes.

## My Brain on Drugs

The phone is ringing in my earbuds. I'm calling Bradley Johnson, the doctor from the Amen Clinic who's going to interpret my brain scan. I'm nervous, but talking to Jim has given me hope. Even if my brain looks like a burnt kernel of popcorn, maybe I can still turn it around.

Dr. Johnson answers and instructs me to open my email. He's sent me my brain scan as well as the scan of a normal, healthy brain, and he wants us to compare them. I put the images up on my computer screen next to each other. It's obvious which is the healthy brain and which is mine. My brain is definitely not perfect. The healthy brain is smooth, with no holes or indentations. Mine looks almost like coral—at least to my untrained eyes. Are there actually holes in my brain? Dr. Johnson assures me that there are not. The scan measures blood flow in the brain, so he can see which areas are more active. From this, he can determine which areas are working well, which are overworked, and which are not working hard enough. The "holes" I see simply indicate low to no metabolic activity. I'm still concerned, especially when he explains there is some possibility that activity can come back. I'd like more assurance than *some* possibility.

Dr. Johnson then directs me to look at my prefrontal cortex, the area in the front of the brain that allows us to make decisions, solve problems, and create plans. This is one of the areas where the visual evidence leaves me most concerned. It looks like two holes have been bored into my frontal lobe, and I wonder if this is what the brain of a lobotomy patient would look like. But Dr. Johnson tells me that the results of the computer spacebar test, the one I was sure I failed, correlate with the image on this scan. People with brains that look like mine and with poor scores on the spacebar test tend to have some degree of attention deficit disorder (ADD). He asks me if I'm easily distractible. Yes. Fidgety? Yep. The "holes" aren't nearly as negative as I feared. There's actually a positive to a brain like mine, he tells me: I'm probably able to sustain periods of prolonged and intense focus. He's right. If something interests me, I can dive in so deep that I shut out any noise or distraction. It's a constant point of contention with Annmarie, because if she asks me a question when I'm in this state, I'll answer but later have no recollection of our conversation. Dr. Johnson also tells me that ADD tends to be more prevalent among very successful people, and therefore it's not always something we should seek to "improve."

I ask him to compare my prefrontal cortex to that of a normal brain. He explains that people with normal brains have a broader range of concentration, but they're not necessarily able to hyperfocus. Their ability to concentrate is more consistent but not as deep.

I consider this a win. So I mark down the score. Kevin's brain: 1. Healthy brain: 0.

Dr. Johnson then moves on to three other aspects of my brain. He starts with the surface of my brain, which isn't as smooth as the healthy brain's. He asks me about my past drug and alcohol use. It's possible that this is why my brain looks this way. It doesn't mean my brain is damaged, he says, but I start to wonder. If my drug and alcohol use caused these changes in the brain, what would it look like after 10 or 15 years of heavy drug use? Almost on cue, Dr. Johnson emails me the scan of an unnamed man with 15-plus years of drug and alcohol abuse. I feel a little better when I see it. His brain is deeply scalloped. Mine isn't even close. Even so, I've got to give a point to the healthy, substance-free brain. Kevin's brain: 1. Healthy brain: 1.

Dr. Johnson shifts focus to the areas of low metabolic activity on the top of my brain.

"Have you ever hit your head?"

"No."

"How about infection? Any long-term infection?"

"Yes, I had Lyme disease."

We must consider that the Lyme disease may be intermittently active, he says. This is one reason why it's such a dreaded infection, as it can linger in the body and flare up well after you think you've vanquished it. This concerns me. They've seen decreased brain function in the scans of people with long-term infections.

I then remember that, in fact, I did hit my head in that spot, almost ten years ago. I was working at a hardware store, delivering rock salt for the winter, and as I picked up a 50-pound bag of salt, I slammed the top of my head into the loading dock. An hour later I was in the emergency room with tunnel vision. I tell him about this.

Again, Dr. Johnson says he can't be sure this is the reason there's low metabolic activity, but it's a possibility. I like him. His thoughtful answers let me know that he's not jumping to conclusions. Kevin's brain: 1. Healthy, never-been-walloped brain: 2.

The final image Dr. Johnson interprets is one that was attached to the initial email. It shows something shaped like a brain crisscrossed with blue lines. There are two patches of red and white. Dr. Johnson tells me that one patch indicates activity in my thalamus, the brain's traffic conductor, which routes motor and sensory signals from body parts to the brain and vice versa. It also regulates wakefulness and sleep. The other colored patch is my cerebellum, the area that coordinates balance, posture, and motor skills. The activity here is slightly lower than in a healthy male brain.

Dr. Johnson tells me that my brain activity should be the other way around—higher in the cerebellum and lower in the thalamus. "This is usually a sign of physical or mental stresses that have been happening long enough to cause physical manifestations," he explains. He then asks about my emotional well-being. I tell him I generally feel great with occasional the-sky-is-collapsing-on-me moments. At such times, I'm generally a ball of anxiety for a day, then back to normal. He says that many people feel this way but also mentions some of the symptoms that someone with brain activity like mine might be feeling: low energy or moodiness. As much as I want to fight it, the doctor is right. I've been pretty stressed lately. Building and managing two businesses, being the best husband and father I can be, and traveling almost nonstop for the past three months have worn me down.

Kevin's brain: 1. Healthy, never injured, never upset, perfect father, homebody brain: 3.

After the phone call, Dr. Johnson sends me a list of the Amen Clinic's recommendations for improving the sea sponge above my shoulders. (My description, not theirs.) Even though I'm down two in the brain department, I now have the cheat sheet to see if I can improve enough to beat out the healthy brain—or at least have a hard time distinguishing between the two.

## BRAIN SUPPLEMENTS AND NUTRIENTS

You don't have to rely on supplements to keep your brain sharp, when there are simple exercises that do the trick. However, here are some supplements the Amen Clinic recommends for brain health, plus a few I've researched and found to be effective.

**Sage.** You might not expect this aromatic herb to have much use beyond your Thanksgiving stuffing, but several studies have found it can improve memory and cognitive functioning, even in people with Alzheimer's disease. Sage acts in a similar way to FDA-approved drugs for Alzheimer's, inhibiting an enzyme that breaks down acetylcholine, a neurotransmitter that's critical for memory, learning, and reasoning.[5]

**Water Hyssop (aka Brahmi, Bacopa).** Long used in Ayurveda, the ancient Indian medical system, this herb with many names is reputed to heal inflammation, joint pain, and skin problems. Modern medical researchers have found that it aids memory as well; recent studies show that it helps us retain new information.

**Acetyl-L-Carnitine (ALC).** ALC is the biologically active amino acid that transports fatty acids from the food we eat to the mitochondria, the tiny "batteries" that produce the energy our cells need to function. Many studies show that ALC can prevent the deterioration of brain cells, thus improving mood and cognition. People who take it regularly report improved memory and heightened alertness.

**Gingko Biloba.** This supplement comes from the oldest tree species on the planet and has long been used in traditional Chinese medicine to enhance memory. Though a few recent studies seem to disprove its benefits, quite a few more studies support the benefits.

**Huperzine.** Extracted from the herb Chinese club moss, huperzine has been found to improve cognitive function in Alzheimer's patients.

**Resveratrol.** Found in the skin of red grapes and berries—not to mention in red wine—resveratrol increases blood flow to the brain. It provides anti-aging benefits and offers protection against Alzheimer's.

**Rosemary.** Recent studies show that rosemary enhances memory and cognitive performance. No wonder it's said that students in ancient Greece used it as a study aid.

With the knowledge we have about health these days, it would be foolish not to incorporate all the techniques you can into your lifestyle to stack the deck in your favor and increase your odds of a longer life. That includes seizing every opportunity to keep your brain sharp, young, and curious.

Jim Kwik says there are two times of life when people experience the most mental decline: when they graduate from school and when they retire. What happens at these times is that people stop being curious. So the key to great brain health, and very possibility to longevity, may be painfully simple: keep learning and keep working.

My grandfather passed away peacefully on May 3, 2014. He certainly would have agreed with Kwik's advice. Learning and working were two of the only constants in the 95 years of his ever-changing life.

# CONCLUSION

## A PERFECT OUTCOME

Over the last 233 days, I've been away from home for 85. I've eaten dinner out probably more than half of the last 233 nights. I've exercised no more than four times a week at best, less than once a week for a few stretches. I've eaten a few pieces of birthday cake. I've had my fair share of wine. I've had moments of binge eating on chips and guacamole. Some people would say I haven't exactly been perfect.

I disagree.

I weighed myself this morning with clothes on, just to be fair to my weight from the beginning, and the scale registered 190 pounds. I've lost a total of 33 pounds, not through some crazy diet but by living my life. I've never once felt deprived. This, to me, *is* perfection.

There were times when I gained two to four pounds over a two-week period of traveling or spending time with family, who like a bit more wine than most Sardinians would recommend. But I'm here now, three belt-buckle notches thinner. My fitness, too, has improved significantly. I've focused on running this entire time—I canceled my gym membership after four trips—and yesterday, I did my four-mile loop in just under 30 minutes, traffic lights included. That's a 7:30 mile. I've also had 225 green smoothies for breakfast. That's been the thing I've done most consistently since the beginning. I missed only a few days because of travel and one-day water fasts.

I'm not a superman. If I had done everything perfectly by objective standards—had less wine and more salad, made dinner at home every night, completely cut out carbs—I'm sure I could have lost 40 or more pounds. If I'd trained five or six times a week, I could have gotten my running time down to under six minutes a mile. I could have gained more muscle. But none of that was my intention. If I'd done all that, I wouldn't have shown myself that my theory of balancing healthy things and things I don't want to give up is actually possible.

It is. I'm proof.

During this time, I've learned a few things I didn't mention in the previous chapters. The first thing I learned is that the little things do count, and the biggest little thing I did was replace my breakfast with a green smoothie. I believe this to be the most powerful, underappreciated secret to not only losing weight but also getting a healthy heap of nutrients into your body before you leave the house in the morning. Victoria Boutenko, author of *Green for Life,* did a small study in which she had 27 people drink a green smoothie every morning for 30 days. This was the only thing in their diet that she asked them to change. After 30 days, the group experienced benefits ranging from weight loss, lower blood pressure, and lower cholesterol to better sleep and improved sex drive.

A green smoothie in the morning works not only because of the nutrients and fiber from the fruits and vegetables but also because of the psychological effect it has on you for the rest of the day. If you have bacon and eggs in the morning, the rest of your day you make bacon-and-eggs eating decisions. But if you have a green smoothie in the morning, the rest of your day is filled with green-smoothie eating decisions. Sounds strange, and it isn't something I can prove. I can only say that you have to experience it for yourself. There's no need for me to load you up with smoothie recipes. Just search *green smoothie recipes* on Google, and you'll have more than you could ever try in a lifetime.

Over the last 233 days, I've also embraced the fact that exercise doesn't work by a one-to-one formula. It's not just about burning more calories than you take in. Of course you burn calories when you exercise. But the *eat-a-calorie, burn-a-calorie* equation fails to take into account that your body becomes more or less efficient at fat burning, depending on your overall state of health. A healthy person burns calories more efficiently than someone in poor health and is likely to have better oxygen uptake, a lower heart rate, lower blood pressure, lower blood sugar, and lower triglycerides (fat in the blood). Focusing on calories alone in your health and fitness regimen is like worrying about the almost empty tank of gas in a car you're driving with three flat tires. The bigger picture is more important.

And the last thing I've really taken to heart in the past 233 days is that it's essential to focus on long-term results. The research my team and I did for this book hammered home the idea that much of our scientific literature comes from an American mind-set of *faster is better.* Yes, you can lose weight faster with high-intensity training, but at what expense? Injury? More stress on the body? Inability to keep up the pace and, eventually, guilt that you failed?

For my own health, I've now adopted a philosophy I borrowed from the Q'ero. When they make decisions they do so with a 1,000-year outlook. This means they ask themselves how they think this decision will play out not in a few weeks or months but in a millennium. This type of future pacing allows them to weigh the time-amplified positives and negatives of their choices.

For my own health, I've now adapted this thinking to my own 100-year outlook. *What will this decision look like for my health in 100 years?* is a very different question than *How can I fit into this dress or these pants in three months?*

Thinking long-term does two things for you and your psyche. First, it takes the pressure off you. Right now, I could be angry that I didn't hit my goal of 185 pounds by the end of August, but what good would that do? What if I make my goal in December? Wouldn't that be cool, too? With a 100-year plan, three or four months don't matter anymore. As long as you're working to improve, you're always winning.

Then, too, thinking into the future like this focuses your mind on doing things that will increase longevity, not on doing things that will put your health in jeopardy simply to reach your short-term goals. You could easily fast for 21 days straight and reach a weight-loss goal, but clearly you wouldn't create a habit of healthy eating during that time. You would learn how to purge. Next up? Binge.

Think like a Q'ero and your body and mind will respond with more patience, better health, and, chances are, longer life.

So, how do I sum all this up and give it a useful context? When I work through my own health challenges now, I look at what I do in four steps:

**Step 1: Assess.** See where you are. Many people just jump into a nutrition or exercise plan without establishing a baseline. Then they never know if they really did themselves any good. If you're taking vitamin D supplements, how do you know if they're helping unless you know what your vitamin D levels were beforehand?

This is the reason I put so much emphasis on blood testing. If you know where you are, you can make informed decisions that will take you where you want to go.

**Step 2: Detox.** Once you've identified a health issue you want to address, it usually requires some sort of detoxification process. Heavy-metal toxicity may require chelation. Too much Internet may require an Internet fast. Overall low energy may require a juice fast.

The detox period is never long-term. It's a 1- to 30-day temporary change that will allow your body to cleanse and reset. Mentally, detox is generally the hardest part of getting well, but when you're done, you almost always feel better and make better decisions.

**Step 3: Retox.** Retox happens as you live your life. Retox occurs when you're at a friend's house for dinner, and you have an extra glass or three of wine. Retox occurs when you're traveling and eat Tex-Mex in Austin for four nights in a row. Retox *is always going to happen*— even if you're in a moment or decade of complete dietary purity. And when it does, just do your best and stay cool. You'll eventually get back on track. That's what Step 4 will help you do.

**Step 4: Repeat.** This is how you improve. You just don't stop after going through Steps 1 to 3 once. You have a 100-year plan, remember? The mind-set around *repeat* is that once you assess, detox, and retox, you'll go through this entire process again. What you'll find is that much of it is the same, but your retox will be different. So the next time, your four nights of Tex-Mex become two. The one-to-three glasses of wine turn into a glass of water (or two glasses of wine and a glass of water). When there's always another chance, your mind does something funny: it makes the process less stressful. Wouldn't it be great if your health weren't another stressor in your life?

So there you have it: my philosophy on getting healthy and living a life you want to live. I hope I've given you ample tools you can use to be happier and healthier, and to stack the longevity deck in your favor. I look forward to hearing about your success.

But I also assure you, your journey is not over. You'll read more books. Find more things to try. Some will work. Some won't. You'll gain weight. You'll lose it. You'll travel, and your diet will unravel. You'll stay home, and it won't. You'll eat out and eat in. All this will happen, and when it does, there's no need to worry. I'll be right there with you—trying some new diet, searching for a lost healing practice in a rainforest halfway around the world, or doing some experimental treatment. Who knows, maybe we'll run into each other at a quiet café in Sardinia and share a bottle of Cannonau wine together.

All I know is that the people who see the search for great health as an adventure are the happiest and the best to be around. So let's do it together—make the search fun and, of course, make it last as long as we can.

# APPENDIX

## THE KALE AND COFFEE
## 21-DAY JUMPSTART

What I'm about to share with you is almost exactly what I did during the first 21 days of my own weight loss. There are some things that I was already doing that I've obviously included here, since I'm assuming that some of you may not already be doing them. If you are already doing them, you can skip them or keep on as you are.

The purpose of this jumpstart is to give you a chance to see just how powerful a few adjustments to your diet and health can actually be. The good news is that at the end, you'll be doing almost exactly what I've done for the past 233 days. I think you'll find that this way of living isn't that difficult and is actually quite fulfilling on all levels. You'll also feel amazing.

This jumpstart is divided into two paths: Easy and Renegade. The easy action? Well, it's easy to do—a great first step. The renegade action is for those of you who are ready to take the plunge. Every day, it's up to you which path you take, so don't feel like you have to stick with easy or renegade all the way through. You can switch it up from day to day. Just be sure to take action and stay with it. It's only for 21 days.

After the first five days, this way of being healthy is probably going to seem easy to you. It may even seem like you're not doing enough. This is on purpose. If you're going to make a lifetime of this, you'd better enjoy it. And if you're still having a problem with feeling like you're getting off too easy, think about all the other plans you've tried that hurt like hell—that worked at first, then brought you right back to being unhappy again.

Let's get going . . .

## Day 1

To start, it's always important to gather data, to set an objective, and to look at where you are now so you can look back and compare later. This is assess mode.

**Easy:** Open a notebook or a new document on your computer and write down some of your current metrics. I'd recommend noting your weight, maybe some measurements, and anything else you're trying to track. If you want to take a "before" picture, that's cool, too. When you revisit this photo after the 21 days, you might be inspired to keep going with the steps you've taken in the Jumpstart.

**Renegade:** In addition to the steps in the Easy track, before Day 1, I'd recommend finding a functional medicine doctor (or going to your existing one, if you have one) to get a full panel of blood tests. Use the list from Chapter 4, and take any additional tests that your health practitioner suggests.

## Day 2

If you're going to jumpstart, you might as well do the hardest part first: the initial detox. There are both biochemical and psychological reasons to start with a detox. The biochemical reason is that a detox will give your body a break almost immediately, so it can start to reset itself. The psychological reason is that after three days of detox, you're likely to see a difference in the way you look and feel, so you'll be more motivated to stick with the rest of this Jumpstart.

**Easy:** For three days, choose either a juice fast, a smoothie fast, or, if you like structure, our Weekend Cleanse program (www.RenegadeHealth. com/weekendcleanse), which is, fittingly, designed to take three days. For a juice fast or smoothie fast, if you don't want to figure it out as you go, you can search online and find plenty of fasts to choose from. Just search *3-day juice fast* or *3-day juice detox* on Google. (Substitute *smoothie* for *juice* if you prefer.) Either plan will work. This is not about doing it "right" by making sure you get the exact amount of nutrition in your body; it's about doing something that gives your body a break.

**Renegade:** The same as Easy. For a deeper cleanse, consider doing one day of water fasting (but only one, and not if you're a type 1 diabetic). Fast with juice or smoothies on the other two days.

## Day 3

This is the second day of whatever cleanse you've chosen. Listed below are some things that I do and don't want you to do during this cleanse.

**Easy:** Do not work hard. Do not be too active. Do not work out. Do relax. Do read a book. Do stay off the computer. Do sleep.

**Renegade:** Same as Easy.

## Day 4

This is the last day of the cleanse you've picked.

**Easy:** Today, continue to enjoy the fact that your body is thankful you're giving it a break. Dine in tonight with your glass of juice or smoothie to celebrate.

**Renegade:** Same as Easy.

## DAY 5

Today, you start drinking green smoothies for the rest of the Jumpstart. Again, I think drinking a green smoothie every day may be the simplest and most effective thing you can do to give yourself a health and longevity edge. If you're totally averse to anything green, try spinach or lettuce in your smoothie: they're the easiest greens to mask with sweet-tasting fruits and berries.

**Easy:** Start your morning green smoothie routine. You don't need to do anything else today except notice how you feel.

Here's my favorite green smoothie recipe, which you can make in a blender.

- 1 head of romaine or red leaf lettuce (½ if it's big)
- One bag of frozen sweet fruit (mangos, apples, or bananas)
- One bag of frozen cherries or berries
- 2 tablespoons of organic hemp seed or 2 scoops of plant protein powder (I like Sun Warrior's Warrior Blend)

**Renegade:** Same as Easy.

## DAY 6

Today is the day to take inventory and start making small changes. You might already be at the next level in some of these, so if you are, devote today to looking around and seeing where you can upgrade what you eat and drink.

**Easy:** Start your day with a green smoothie. Take a look at the salt you use, wine you drink, coffee you drink, and meat you eat. Pick one and decide to upgrade it.

- For salt, consider switching to Aztec Sea Salt or Celtic Sea Salt.

- For wine, try Frog's Leap.

- For coffee, try Bulletproof.

- Get quality organic, grass-finished meat at your local butcher shop.

**Renegade:** Upgrade all of the above.

## Day 7

This is the first day of your stress-free (or maybe less stressed) life. After today, you'll be armed with two effective stress-relief tools to use as needed.

**Easy:** Start your day with a green smoothie. Go to your local health food store and get holy basil (or order it online). Take one hour and watch this video on how to tap (www.RenegadeHealth.com/tappingvideo) and then tap for 15 minutes on something that is causing you anxiety. You can always find tapping scripts on Google. Just search *Tapping script for [your issue]*.

**Renegade:** Same as Easy.

## Day 8

Today is the first of four food-elimination days. The first food you're going to take out of your diet for the next seven days is sugar. From today until Day 15, no sugar will pass your lips. This will help recalibrate your body to react to sugar as it should. If your diet now includes sugar, chances are your body has built up a tolerance for it that may not be good for you.

**Easy:** Start your day with a green smoothie. No sugar until Day 15. No candy, no honey, no agave, no sweetened drinks. You can eat fruit.

**Renegade:** Same as Easy.

## Day 9

Today is the second food-elimination day. No caffeine for the next seven days. This will give your adrenals a chance to reset. You may be tired and have a headache the first few days without caffeine. Stick with it. You won't have to quit forever, just for the next week.

**Easy:** Start your day with a green smoothie. No caffeine until Day 16. No coffee, no green tea, no chocolate, no maté. You can drink herbal teas or holy basil tea.

**Renegade:** Same as Easy.

## Day 10

Today is your third food-elimination day. No wheat or soy for a week. These are two common allergens that many people have trouble eating. We're going to take them out of your diet for seven days and then bring them back to see how you feel when you eat them again.

**Easy:** Start your day with a green smoothie. No wheat or soy until Day 17.

**Renegade:** Same as Easy. If you want to dig deeper, go to www. RenegadeHealth.com/glutentest and order a gluten gene test.

## DAY 11

Today is the last food-elimination day. No dairy for a week. Cut it out completely and see how you feel.

**Easy:** Start your day with a green smoothie. No dairy until Day 18. No cheese, no milk, no butter, no cream, no yogurt.

**Renegade:** Same as Easy.

## DAY 12

All this talk about food—but none about exercise? Finally, today you're going to start an experiment. You're going to start checking your heart rate to see what it is when you exercise.

**Easy:** Before you get out of bed, find your resting heart rate, using the process I outlined on page 90. Next, start your day with a green smoothie. Sometime today, find 30 minutes to do your regular workout. If you don't exercise, walk for that same amount of time. Every five minutes during your workout, check your heart rate just as you did in the morning. After you're finished exercising, use your resting heart rate to calculate your fat-burning heart rate, with Phil Maffetone's 180 Formula (www.philmaffetone.com/180-formula). Compare your fat-burning rate to the heart rate you reached during your workout to see if it was close, over, or under.

**Renegade:** Same as Easy. If you don't want to check your heart rate manually, you can buy a heart rate monitor. There are plenty of good ones available. I like the kind that connects to my smartphone.

## DAY 13

Do a media fast. Today's the day that you begin a seven-day break from the media. Yep, that's just about everything: no TV, no Internet news sites, no newspapers, no social media for the next week. You can read books or watch documentaries during this time, but that's the only information you can immerse yourself in. (If you happen to work in the media or you're required to use media for your job, skip this step for now and do it on your next week-long vacation.)

**Easy:** Start your day with a green smoothie, without your morning paper or smartphone check-in. Download SelfRestraint for PC or SelfControl for Mac. These programs will block the websites of your choice for a period of time that you determine—one, two, five, ten hours. Today, and for the next seven days, until Day 20, block all your favorite websites, including social media websites.

**Renegade:** Do the above, but also cancel your cable TV. Seriously. Do it. You won't miss it.

## DAY 14

Today, you're going to train in your fat-burning heart rate zone. Two days ago, you found out the heart rate at which you normally train, but now you're going to either train a little harder, if your heart rate wasn't up to your fat-burning zone, or train lighter, if you exceeded it.

**Easy:** Start your day with a green smoothie. Today take 30 to 45 minutes to train in your fat-burning heart rate zone. Check your heart rate every five to seven minutes to see if you're there.

**Renegade:** Same as Easy. Plus, buy Phil Maffetone's book *The Maffetone Method* and Danny Dreyer's *ChiRunning* or *ChiWalking* to read when the Jumpstart is done.

## Day 15

Reintroduction day: Sugar.

**Easy:** Start your day with a green smoothie. Reintroduce sugar if you want and see how you feel. If you don't want to, that's cool, too. Keep abstaining until you feel like you're done and want to reintroduce it.

**Renegade:** Same as Easy. Consider this the time to remove any nonfruit sugar from your diet long-term, and eat it only as a treat.

## Day 16

Reintroduction day: Caffeine.

**Easy:** Start your day with a green smoothie. Reintroduce caffeine if you want and see how you feel. If you don't want to, that's cool, too. Keep abstaining until you feel like you're done and want to reintroduce it. If possible, try a coffee like Bulletproof or Longevity. If you prefer green tea, consider trying one of the two I found that are lower in lead: Choice Organic Premium Japanese Green Tea (grown in Brazil) or Japanese Kukicha Kabuse Green Tea Leaf, Organic.

**Renegade:** Same as Easy.

## Day 17

Reintroduction day: Wheat and soy.

**Easy:** Start your day with a green smoothie. Reintroduce wheat if you want and see how you feel. If you don't want to, that's cool, too. Keep abstaining until you feel like you're done and want to reintroduce it. Consider not reintroducing soy at all. Soy can interfere with your hormones. Also, most of the soy available in the United States is genetically modified. I do not consider the soy on the market today a health food and would eat it extremely sparingly, or not at all.

**Renegade:** Same as Easy. Also consider eating a low- to no-gluten diet for as long as you feel comfortable.

## Day 18

Reintroduction day: Dairy.

**Easy:** Start your day with a green smoothie. Reintroduce dairy if you want and see how you feel. If you don't want to, that's cool, too. Keep abstaining until you feel like you're done and want to reintroduce it. When you do reintroduce dairy, I'd suggest organic products from goat's milk or sheep's milk. They're easier to digest than cow's milk products.

**Renegade:** Same as Easy. If you feel inclined, keep up your dairy-free experiment for a few more weeks and see how you feel.

## Day 19

Today is a stress check-in day. You've already done one day of tapping, on Day 7, so today, do another 30 minutes.

**Easy:** Start your day with a green smoothie. Sometime today, take 30 minutes and do a few rounds of tapping on either the same issue you were dealing with on Day 7 or something completely different. If you haven't ordered holy basil yet, now's the time to do it. Here's a link if you want to try ours: www.RenegadeHealth.com/holybasil.

**Renegade:** Same as above.

## Day 20

Your media fast is over!

**Easy:** Start your day with a green smoothie, then go back to your Facebook updates, TMZ, and Gawker. Just kidding. Try to ease back into media, especially social media. Chances are you didn't miss much.

**Renegade:** Same as Easy. Did you cancel your cable?

## Day 21

Celebrate. You did it!

Today, the only thing I ask you to do is spend 15 minutes with yourself and think about what in your life you would change if you had a 100-year plan for your health. Write them down. Over the next few months and years, start adjusting those areas of your life to fit your new long-term plan.

If you like, you can take an "after" picture and compare it to your "before" shot from Day 1! If you want to send us the photos and tell us about your experience doing the 21-Day Jumpstart, that would be awesome. Just head over to www.RenegadeHealth.com or www.KevinGianni.com and drop me a line.

# ENDNOTES

## Chapter 2  How My 15 Minutes of Fame Could Screw Up Your Quest for 90-Plus Years of Life

1.  Federal Trade Commission, "FTC Investigation of Ad Claims that Rice Krispies Benefits Children's Immunity Leads to Stronger Order Against Kellogg," FTC Docket No. C-4262, press release issued June 3, 2010, http://www.ftc.gov/news-events/press-releases/2010/06/ftc-investigation-ad-claims-rice-krispies-benefits-childrens.

2.  Ibid.

3.  Ibid.

4.  Paul Pestano et al., "Sugar in Children's Cereals: Popular Brands Pack More Sugar than Snack Cakes and Cookies," Environmental Working Group, November 20, 2011, http://www.foodpolitics.com/wp-content/uploads/CEREALSewg_press_cereal_report.pdf.

## Chapter 3  The Dubious Distinction of Being the Only Animal on the Planet That Doesn't Know What to Eat

1.  Paignton Zoo Park, "Taking Diet Tips from Monkeys," newsletter, January 14, 2014, http://www.paigntonzoo.org.uk/news/details/taking-diet-tips-from-monkeys.

2.  Consumer Reports Food Safety and Sustainability Center, "Executive Summary," in *Report on Corn and Soy in GMOs,* October 2014, http://www.greenerchoices.org/pdf/CR_FSASC_GMO_Final_Report_10062014.pdf.

3.  Alberto Finamore et al., "Intestinal and Peripheral Immune Response to MON810 Maize Ingestion in Weaning and Old Mice," *Journal of Agriculture and Food*

*Chemistry* 56, no. 23 (2008): 11533, http://www.cyberacteurs.org/sans_ogm/fichiers/finamore08-jf802059w.pdf.

4.  Dan Buettner, *The Blue Zones: 9 Lessons for Living Longer from the People Who've Lived the Longest,* 2nd ed. (Washington, D.C.: National Geographic, 2012).

5.  Michael Pollan, *In Defense of Food: An Eater's Manifesto* (New York: Penguin, 2009): 146.

## Chapter 4   How a Horny Hog Could Be the Key to Your Longevity

1.  The Weston Price Foundation. http://www.westonaprice.org/about-the-foundation/about-us/.

2.  "The (Not So) Secret Life of Our Inner Neanderthal," *Science in the News,* May 19, 2014, http://sitn.hms.harvard.edu/flash/2014/the-not-so-secret-life-of-our-inner-neanderthal/.

## Chapter 5   My Contaminated Kitchen Cabinet: A Surprising Result

1.  "Cadmium: Safety and Health Topics," Occupational Safety & Health Administration (OSHA), United States Department of Labor, https://www.osha.gov/SLTC/cadmium/. Accessed January 27, 2015.

2.  Environmental Working Group, "Body Burden: The Pollution in Newborns," July 14, 2005, http://www.ewg.org/research/body-burden-pollution-newborns/.

3.  "Fourth National Report on Human Exposure to Environmental Chemicals," Department of Health and Human Resources, Centers for Disease Control and Prevention, 2009, http://www.cdc.gov/exposurereport/pdf/fourthreport.pdf.

4.  Bryan Walsh, "The Perils of Plastic," *Time,* April 1, 2010, http://content.time.com/time/specials/packages/article/0,28804,1976909_1976908,00.html.

5.  Marian Burros, "High Mercury Levels Are Found in Tuna Sushi," *The New York Times,* January 23, 2008, http://www.nytimes.com/2008/01/23/dining/23sushi.html?pagewanted=all.

6.  "2007 New York City Department of Health and Mental Hygiene (DOHMH) Health Advisory #11: Blood Mercury Levels in NYC Adult Women Are Higher Than Women Nationally; Providers Should Encourage Healthy Fish Consumption," City of New York Department of Health and Mental Hygiene, http://www.nyc.gov/html/doh/downloads/pdf/lead/mercury_advisory11_72307.pdf.

7.  American Congress of Obstetricians and Gynecologists, "Exposure to Environmental Toxins and Agents," Committee Opinion No. 595, October 2013, https://

www.acog.org/Resources-And-Publications/Committee-Opinions/Committee-on-Health-Care-for-Underserved-Women/Exposure-to-Toxic-Environmental-Agents.

8. National Institute of Environmental Health Services, "Bisphenol A," http://www.niehs.nih.gov/health/topics/agents/sya-bpa/.

9. Chun Z. Yang et al., "Most Plastic Products Release Estrogenic Chemicals: A Potential Health Problem That Can Be Solved," *Environmental Health Perspectives* 119, no. 7 (July 1, 2011), http://www.ncbi.nlm.nih.gov/pmc/articles/PMC3222987/.

10. Erica Gies, "Substitutes for Bisphenol A Could Be More Harmful," *The New York Times,* April 18, 2011, http://www.nytimes.com/2011/04/18/business/global/18iht-rbog-plastic-18.html.

11. "What Is BPA (Bisphenol A)? Is BPA Harmful?" *Medical News Today,* last modified September 26, 2014, http://www.medicalnewstoday.com/articles/221205.php.

12. David Markell, "An Overview of TSCA, Its History and Key Underlying Assumptions, and Its Place in Environmental Regulation," *Washington University Journal of Law and Policy* 32 (2010): 352, http://openscholarship.wustl.edu/cgi/viewcontent.cgi?article=1084&context=law_journal_law_policy.

13. Ken Cook, Environmental Working Group, *10 Americans,* YouTube, last modified July 23, 2012, https://www.youtube.com/watch?v=0-kc3AIM_LU.

14. Chemical Safety Improvement Act, S. 1009, 113th Congress (2013–2015), https://www.congress.gov/bill/113th-congress/senate-bill/1009.

15. Ken Cook, *10 Americans.*

## Chapter 6   The Curious Thing about Eating Animals (an Ex-Vegan Perspective)

1. "Kings of the Carnivores," *Economist Online,* April 30, 2012, http://www.economist.com/blogs/graphicdetail/2012/04/daily-chart-17.

2. Briana Pobiner, "Evidence for Meat-Eating by Early Humans," *Nature* 4, no. 6 (2013): 1, http://www.nature.com/scitable/knowledge/library/evidence-for-meat-eating-by-early-humans-103874273.

3. James Owen, "Goats Key to Spread of Farming, Gene Study Suggests," *National Geographic News,* October 10, 2006, http://news.nationalgeographic.com/news/2006/10/061010-goats-history.html.

4. Organic Consumers Association, "Disturbing Facts on Factory Farming and Food Safety," http://www.organicconsumers.org/Toxic/factoryfarm.cfm.

5. Michael Pollan, *The Omnivore's Dilemma: A Natural History of Four Meals* (New York: Penguin, 2007): 78.

6. A. J. McAfee et al., "Red Meat from Animals Offered a Grass Diet Increases Plasma and Platelet n-3 PUFA in Healthy Consumers," *British Journal of Nutrition* 105, no. 1 (January 2011): 80–9, http://www.ncbi.nlm.nih.gov/pubmed/20807460.

7. Cynthia A. Daley, "A Review of Fatty Acid Profiles and Antioxidant Content in Grass-Fed and Grain-Fed Beef," *Nutrition Journal* 9, no. 10 (March 10, 2010), http://www.nutritionj.com/content/9/1/10.

8. Toby G. Knowles, "Leg Disorders in Broiler Chickens: Prevalence, Risk Factors, and Prevention," *PLOS One* 3, no. 2 (February 6, 2008), http://www.ncbi.nlm.nih.gov/pmc/articles/PMC2212134.

9. Tom Philpott, "The Meat Industry Now Consumes Four-Fifths of All Antibiotics," *Mother Jones,* February 8, 2013, http://www.motherjones.com/tom-philpott/2013/02/meat-industry-still-gorging-antibiotics.

10. David G. White, "The Isolation of Antibiotic-Resistant Salmonella from Retail Ground Meats," *New England Journal of Medicine* 345 (October 18, 2001): 1147–54, http://www.nejm.org/doi/full/10.1056/NEJMoa010315.

11. Daan Kromhout, "Serum Cholesterol in Cross-Cultural Perspective: The Seven Countries Study," *Acta Cardiologica* 54, no. 3 (1999): 155–8, http://www.ncbi.nlm.nih.gov/pubmed/10478272. See also The Seven Countries Study official website, http://sevencountriesstudy.com.

12. Dariush Mozaffarian et al., "Fish Intake, Contaminants, and Human Health: Evaluating the Risks and the Benefits," *Journal of the American Medical Association* 296, no. 15 (2006): 1885–99, http://jama.jamanetwork.com/article.aspx?articleid=203640.

13. Ibid.

14. Cyrus A. Raji et al., "Regular Fish Consumption and Age-Related Brain Gray Matter," *American Journal of Preventive Medicine,* July 29, 2014, http://www.ajpmonline.org/article/S0749-3797(14)00257-8/abstract.

15. Carmen Cavada and Wolfram Schultz, "The Mysterious Orbitofrontal Cortex. Foreword," *Cerebral Cortex* 10, no. 3 (2000), http://cercor.oxfordjournals.org/content/10/3/205.full.pdf.

16. Environmental Working Group, "First-Ever U.S. Tests of Farmed Salmon Show High Levels of Cancer-Causing PCBs," news release, July 30, 2003, http://www.ewg.org/news/news-releases/2003/07/30/first-ever-us-tests-farmed-salmon-show-high-levels-cancer-causing-pcbs.

17. "Fish: Friend or Foe?" *The Nutrition Source,* Harvard School of Public Health, http://www.hsph.harvard.edu/nutritionsource/fish/.

## Chapter 7  Exercise: Almost Everyone Does It Wrong; Here's How to Do It Right

1.  Marna Rayl Greenberg et al., "Unique Obstacle Race Injuries at an Extreme Sports Event: A Case Series," *Annals of Emergency Medicine* 63, no. 3 (March 2014): 361–6; epub November 18, 2013, http://www.annemergmed.com /article/S0196-0644(13)01481-9/abstract.

2.  Bernd Heinrich, *Why We Run: A Natural History* (New York: Harper Collins, 2002): 177.

3.  Christopher McDougall, *Born to Run: A Hidden Tribe, Superathletes, and the Greatest Race the World Has Never Seen* (New York: Alfred A. Knopf, 2009): 229.

4.  Richard P. Troiano et al., "Physical Activity in the United States Measured by Accelerometer," *Medicine & Science in Sports & Exercise* 40, no. 1 (January 2008): 181–6, http://www.ncbi.nlm.nih.gov/pubmed/18091006.

5.  Centers for Disease Control and Prevention, "One in Five Adults Meet Physical Activity Guidelines," May 2, 2013, http://www.cdc.gov/media/releases/2013/ p0502-physical-activity.html.

6.  Christopher McDougall, "The Once and Future Way to Run," *The New York Times,* November 2, 2011, http://www.nytimes.com/2011/11/06/magazine/ running-christopher-mcdougall.html?pagewanted=all&_r=0.

7.  Benjamin M. Weistenthal et al., "Injury Rates and Patterns among CrossFit Athletes," *Orthopaedic Journal of Sports Medicine* 2, no. 4 (April 25, 2014), http://ojs. sagepub.com/content/2/4/2325967114531177.full.

8.  Christopher McDougall, "The Once and Future Way to Run."

9.  Phil Maffetone, "Revisiting Triathlon after 17 Years: Athletes Are Still Overtraining!" Natural Running Center, July 18, 2012, http://naturalrunningcenter. com/2012/07/18/revisiting-triathlon-athletes-overtraining/.

10. Gretchen Reynolds, *The First Twenty Minutes: Surprising Science Reveals How We Can Exercise Better, Train Smarter, Live Longer* (New York: Plume, 2013): 239.

11. Herbert J. Levine, M.D., "Rest Heart Rate and Life Expectancy," *Journal of the American College of Cardiology* 30, no. 4 (October 1997): 1104–6, http://content. onlinejacc.org/article.aspx?articleid=1124183.

## Chapter 8  How One Crazy Technique and an Herb from India Could Add Years to Your Life

1.  Jason P. Block et al., "Psychosocial Stress and Change in Weight among U.S. Adults," *American Journal of Epidemiology* 170, no. 2 (May 22, 2009): 181–92, http://aje.oxfordjournals.org/content/170/2/181.abstract.

2.  Sheldon Cohen et al., "Chronic Stress, Glucocorticoid Receptor Resistance, Inflammation, and Disease Risk," *Proceedings of the National Academy of Sciences of the United States of America* 109, no. 16 (April 2, 2012), http://www.pnas.org/content/109/16/5995.abstract?tab=author-info.

3.  Carnegie Mellon University, "Stress on Disease," Homepage Stories, http://www.cmu.edu/homepage/health/2012/spring/stress-on-disease.shtml.

4.  Mark Hyman, "Inflammation: How to Cool the Fire Inside You That's Making You Fat and Diseased," last modified January 27, 2012, http://drhyman.com/blog/2012/01/27/inflammation-how-to-cool-the-fire-inside-you-thats-making-you-fat-and-diseased/#close.

5.  Dawson Church et al., "Psychological Trauma Symptom Improvement in Veterans Using Emotional Freedom Techniques: A Randomized Controlled Trial," *Journal of Nervous & Mental Disease* 201 (February 2013): 153–60, http://www.academia.edu/4442547/Psychological_trauma_symptom_improvement_in_veterans_using_EFT_Emotional_Freedom_Techniques_A_randomized_controlled_trial.

6.  Claire Kowalchik and William H. Hylton, eds., *Rodale's Illustrated Encyclopedia of Herbs* (Emmaus, PA: Rodale Books, 1998): 22.

7.  Deni Bown, *New Encyclopedia of Herbs & Their Uses* (New York, DK Publishing, 2001).

8.  Ibid.

9.  Priyabrata Pattanayak et al., "Study 2: *Ocimum sanctum* Linn. A Reservoir Plant for Therapeutic Applications: An Overview," *Pharmacognosy Reviews* 4, no. 7 (January–June 2010): 95–105.

10. Andrew Weil, "Holy Basil to Combat Stress?" Q&A Library, November 5, 2004, http://www.drweil.com/drw/u/QAA346157/holy-basil-to-combat-stress.html.

## Chapter 9    Sugar, Carbs, and Gluten: A Holy Trinity of Disease . . . or Not?

1.  T. Colin Campbell, Ph.D., with Thomas M. Campbell II, M.D., *The China Study: Startling Implications for Diet, Weight Loss, and Long-Term Health* (Dallas, TX: Ben Bella Books, 2004).

2.  Neal D. Barnard et al., "A Low-Fat Vegan Diet Improves Glycemic Control and Cardiovascular Risk Factors in a Randomized Clinical Trial in Individuals with Type 2 Diabetes," *Diabetes Care* 29, no. 8 (August 2006): 1777–83, http://care.diabetesjournals.org/content/29/8/1777.abstract.

3.  "HealthWatch: Caveman Diet Helps Diabetics in UCSF Study," CBS San Francisco, November 7, 2011, http://sanfrancisco.cbslocal.com/2011/11/07/healthwatch-caveman-diet-helps-diabetics-in-ucsf-study/.

4.  Kazuaki Ohtsubo et al., "Pathway to Diabetes Through Attenuation of Pancre-
    atic Beta Cell Glycosylation and Glucose Transport," *Nature Medicine* 17, no. 9
    (August 14, 2011): 1067–75, http://www.nature.com/nm/journal/v17/n9/full/
    nm.2414.html.

5.  Belinda S. Lennerz et al., "Effects of Dietary Glycemic Index on Brain Regions
    Related to Reward and Craving in Men," *American Journal of Clinical Nutri-
    tion* 98, no. 3 (September 2013): 641–7; first published online, June 26,
    2013, http://ajcn.nutrition.org/content/early/2013/06/26/ajcn.113.064113.
    abstract?sid=44ef5031-b040-4501-8e93-af85301d69c6.

6.  Bryan Dowd and John Walker-Smith, "Samuel Gee, Aretaeus, and the Coeliac Af-
    fection," *British Medical Journal* 2 (April 6, 1974): 45–7, http://www.ncbi.nlm.nih.
    gov/pmc/articles/PMC1610148/pdf/brmedj01971-0061.pdf.

7.  Monty S. Losowsky, "A History of Coeliac Disease," *Digestive Diseases* 26, no. 2
    (April 21, 2008): 112–20, http://www.ncbi.nlm.nih.gov/pubmed/18431060.

8.  Kiera Butler, "Is Wheat Gluten Really Bad for Everyone?" *Mother Jones,* February
    7, 2013, http://www.motherjones.com/environment/2013/02/gluten-free-diet-
    fad.

9.  Alberto Rubio-Tapia et al., "Increased Prevalence and Mortality in Undiagnosed
    Celiac Disease," *Gastroenterology* 137, issue 1 (July 2009): 88–93; first published
    online April 13, 2009, http://dx.doi.org/10.1053/j.gastro.2009.03.059.

10. U.S. Dairy Export Council, *Reference Manual for U.S. Whey and Lactose Products,*
    Véronique Lagrange, editor, 3rd. ed. (2008): 66, http://usdec.files.cms-plus.com/
    PDFs/2008ReferenceManuals/Whey_Lactose_Reference_Manual_Complete2_Op-
    timized.pdf.

11. Jessica R. Biesiekierski et al., "Gluten Causes Gastrointestinal Symptoms in Sub-
    jects Without Celiac Disease: A Double-Blind Randomized Placebo-Controlled
    Trial," *American Journal of Gastroenterology* 106, no. 3 (March 2011): 508–14,
    http://www.ncbi.nlm.nih.gov/pubmed/21224837.

12. Jessica R. Biesiekierski et al., "No Effects of Gluten in Patients with Self-Reported
    Non-Celiac Gluten Sensitivity after Dietary Reduction of Fermentable, Poorly Ab-
    sorbed, Short-Chain Carbohydrates," *American Journal of Gastroenterology* 145,
    no. 2 (August 2013): 320-8; first published online May 6, 2013, http://www.
    gastrojournal.org/article/S0016-5085(13)00702-6/abstract.

# Chapter 10   An Interesting Conclusion about Beer, Wine, and Spirits

1.  Jara Pérez-Jiménez et al., "Identification of the 100 Richest Dietary Sources of
    Polyphenols: An Application of the Phenol-Explorer Database," *European Journal
    of Clinical Nutrition* 64 (November 2010): S112–S120, http://www.nature.com/
    ejcn/journal/v64/n3s/fig_tab/ejcn2010221t1.html#t1-fn.

2.  Martinette T. Streppel et al., "Long-Term Wine Consumption Is Related to Cardiovascular Mortality and Life Expectancy Independently of Moderate Alcohol Intake: The Zutphen Study," *Journal of Epidemiology and Community Health* 63, no. 7 (July 2009): 534–40; first published online April 2009, http://jech.bmj.com/content/early/2009/04/30/jech.2008.082198.short?q=w_jech_ahead_tab.

3.  Harvard School of Public Health, "Alcohol and Heart Disease," http://www.hsph.harvard.edu/nutritionsource/alcohol-and-heart-disease/.

4.  K. Ozasa et al., "Alcohol Use and Mortality in the Japan Collaborative Cohort Study for Evaluation of Cancer (JACC)," *Asian Pacific Journal of Cancer Prevention* 8 supplement (2007): 81–8, http://www.ncbi.nlm.nih.gov/pubmed/18260706.

5.  Serge C. Renaud et al., "Wine, Beer, and Mortality in Middle-Aged Men from Eastern France," *Archives of Internal Medicine* 159, no. 16 (September 12, 2009): 1865–70, http://www.ncbi.nlm.nih.gov/pubmed/10493316?dopt=Citation.

6.  Edward J. Neafsey and Michael Collins, "Moderate Alcohol Consumption and Cognitive Risk," *Neuropsychiatric Disease and Treatment* 7, no. 16 (August 2011): 465–84, http://www.dovepress.com/moderate-alcohol-consumption-and-cognitive-risk-peer-reviewed-article-NDT.

7.  F. M. Booyse et al., "Mechanism by Which Alcohol and Wine Polyphenols Affect Coronary Heart Disease Risk," *Annals of Epidemiology* 17, no. 5 (May 2007): S24–S31, http://www.ncbi.nlm.nih.gov/pubmed/17478321?dopt=Citation.

8.  Liam J. Murray et al., "Inverse Relationship Between Alcohol Consumption and Active Helicobacter Pylori Infection: The Bristol Helicobacter Project," *American Journal of Gastroenterology* 97 (2002): 2750–5, http://www.nature.com/ajg/journal/v97/n11/abs/ajg2002707a.html.

9.  National Institute on Alcohol Abuse and Alcoholism, "Drinking Levels Defined," http://www.niaaa.nih.gov/alcohol-health/overview-alcohol-consumption/moderate-binge-drinking.

10. Mayo Clinic, "Alcohol Use: If You Drink, Keep It Moderate," http://www.mayoclinic.org/healthy-living/nutrition-and-healthy-eating/in-depth/alcohol/art-20044551.

11. Lecia Bushak, "A Bottle of Wine a Day Is 'Good for You,' Researchers Say: Why You Need to Be Careful about the Claim," *Medical Daily* (April 24, 2014), http://www.medicaldaily.com/bottle-wine-day-good-you-researchers-say-why-you-need-be-careful-about-claim-278702.

12. Daily Mail Reporter, "Bottle of Wine a Day 'Is Not Bad for You': Leading Scientist Also Claims Those Who Exceed Recommended Dose Could Live Longer than Teetotalers," *Daily Mail.com* (April 19, 2014), http://www.dailymail.co.uk/news/article-2608193/Bottle-wine-day-not-bad-Leading-scientist-claim-exceed-recommended-does-live-longer-teetotallers.html.

13. George A. Bray et al., "Consumption of High-Fructose Corn Syrup in Beverages May Play a Role in the Epidemic of Obesity," *American Journal of Clinical Nutrition* 79, no. 4 (April 2004): 537–43, http://ajcn.nutrition.org/content/79/4/537. short.

## Chapter 11   What an Almost-90-Day Experiment (Binge) Taught Me about America's Most Popular Pick-Me-Up

1.   M. H. Eskelinen et al., "Midlife Coffee and Tea Drinking and the Risk of Late-Life Dementia: A Population-Based CAIDE Study," *Journal of Alzheimer's Disease* 16, no. 2 (2009): 85–91, http://www.ncbi.nlm.nih.gov/pubmed/19158424.

2.   G. W. Ross et al., "Association of Coffee and Caffeine Intake with the Risk of Parkinson Disease," *Journal of the American Medical Association* 283, no. 20 (May 24–31, 2000): 2674–9, http://www.ncbi.nlm.nih.gov/pubmed/10819950.

3.   Chuanhai Cao et al., "High Blood Caffeine Levels in MCI Linked to Lack of Progression to Dementia," *Journal of Alzheimer's Disease* 30 (2012): 559–72, http://health.usf.edu/nocms/publicaffairs/now/pdfs/jad111781.pdf.

4.   Fengju Song et al., "Increased Caffeine Intake Is Associated with Reduced Risk of Basal Cell Carcinoma of the Skin," *Journal of Cancer Research* 72 (July 1, 2012): 3282, http://cancerres.aacrjournals.org/content/72/13/3282.

5.   Celia Hall, "Study Links Coffee to Stiffening of Arteries," September 3, 2001, www.telegraph.co.uk/news/worldnews/europe/greece/1339369/Study-links-coffee-to-stiffening-of-arteries.html.

6.   Mayo Clinic Staff, "Caffeine Content for Coffee, Tea, Soda, and More," http://www.mayoclinic.org/healthy-living/nutrition-and-healthy-eating/in-depth/caffeine/art-20049372.

7.   M. Heliovaara, "Coffee Consumption, Rheumatoid Factor, and the Risk of Rheumatoid Arthritis," *Annals of the Rheumatic Diseases* 59, no. 8 (August 2000): 631–5, http://www.ncbi.nlm.nih.gov/pmc/articles/PMC1753204/.

8.   A. Yang, "Genetics of Caffeine Consumption and Responses to Caffeine," *Pharmapsychology* 211, no. 3 (August 2010): 245–57, http://www.ncbi.nlm.nih.gov/pubmed/20532872.

9.   "The DNA of Thanksgiving," 23andMe.com, http://visual.ly/dna-thanksgiving.

## Chapter 12  Salt: No Good for Slugs, but What about Us?

1.   Natalie Engler, "Marathon Dilemma: How Much Water Is Too Much?" Reuters Health, 2003, http://www.amaasportsmed.org/news_room/hyponatremia_reuters.htm.

2.  Centers for Disease Control and Prevention (CDC), "Americans Consume Too Much Salt," http://www.cdc.gov/features/dssodium/.

3.  Massimo Cirillo et al., "A History of Salt," *American Journal of Nephrology* 14, no. 46 (1994): 426–31, http://www.ncbi.nlm.nih.gov/pubmed/7847480.

4.  "Intersalt: An International Study of Electrolyte Excretion and Blood Pressure. Results for 24 Hour Urinary Sodium and Potassium Excretion. Intersalt Cooperative Research Group," *British Medical Journal* 297, no. 6644 (July 30, 1988): 319–28, http://www.ncbi.nlm.nih.gov/pubmed/3416162.

5.  Melinda Wenner Moyer, "It's Time to End the War on Salt," *Scientific American,* July 8, 2011, http://www.scientificamerican.com/article/its-time-to-end-the-war-on-salt/.

6.  "Sodium (Chloride)," Micronutrient Information Center, Linus Pauling Institute, http://lpi.oregonstate.edu/infocenter/minerals/sodium/.

7.  Swasti Tiwari, "Insulin's Impact on Renal Sodium Transport and Blood Pressure in Health, Obesity, and Diabetes," *American Journal of Physiology* 293, no. 4 (October 1, 2007), http://ajprenal.physiology.org/content/293/4/F974.

8.  "Introduction of Iodized Salt in the 1920's Linked to Increased IQ and Growth in the U.S. and Switzerland," *IDD Newsletter,* August 2013, http://www.iccidd.org/newsletter/idd_aug13_growth_and_iq.pdf.

## Chapter 13   Need More Energy? Do Nothing. Well, Kind Of . . .

1.  Alan Goldhamer, "Medically Supervised Water-Only Fasting in the Treatment of Hypertension," *Journal of Manipulative and Physiological Therapeutics* 24, no. 5 (June 2001): 335–9, http://www.vegsource.com/articles/goldhamer.pdf.

## Chapter 14   My Entenmann's-Cake-Eating Grandfather Shows Me The Last Secret of the Longest-Lived People

1.  Qiuping Gu et al., "Prescription Drug Use Continues to Increase: U.S. Prescription Drug Data for 2007–2008," Centers for Disease Control and Prevention, NCHS Data Brief no. 42, September 2010, http://www.cdc.gov/nchs/data/databriefs/db42.htm.

2.  Gina Kolata, "Live Long? Die Young? Answer Isn't Just in Genes," *The New York Times,* August 31, 2006, http://www.nytimes.com/2006/08/31/health/31age.html?pagewanted=all&_r=1&.

3.  Riccardo E. Marioni et al., "Active Cognitive Lifestyle Is Associated with Positive Cognitive Health Transitions and Compression of Morbidity from Age Sixty-Five," *PLOS ONE,* no. 12 (December 12, 2012), http://www.plosone.org/article/info%3Adoi%2F10.1371%2Fjournal.pone.0050940.

4.   David A. Snowdon, "Healthy Aging and Dementia: Findings from the Nun Study," *Annals of Internal Medicine* 139, no. 5, pt. 2 (September 2, 2003): 450–4.

5.   Shahin Akhondzadeh et al., "*Salvia officinalis* Extract in the Treatment of Patients with Mild to Moderate Alzheimer's Disease: A Double-Blind, Randomized, and Placebo-controlled Trial," *Journal of Clinical Pharmacy and Therapeutics* 28, no. 1 (February 2003): 53–9, http://www.ncbi.nlm.nih.gov/pubmed/12605619; Nicola T.J. Tildesley et al., "*Salvia lavandulaefolia* (Spanish Sage) Enhances Memory in Healthy Young Volunteers," *Pharmacology Biochemistry and Behavior* 75, issue 3 (June 2003): 669–74, http://www.sciencedirect.com/science/article/pii/S0091305703001229; Andrew B. Scholey et al., "An Extract of Salvia (Sage) with Anticholinesterase Properties Improves Memory and Attention in Healthy Older Volunteers," *Psychopharmacology* 198, no. 1 (May 2008): 127–39, http://www.ncbi.nlm.nih.gov/pubmed/18350281.

# ACKNOWLEDGMENTS

Books are hard to write and are never completed alone. There were many involved in this process I'd like to thank.

My wife, Annmarie, the most patient, loving, and understanding person I've ever met. Anyone who can spend two and a half years with me in less than 300 square feet is more than special. This book would never have happened if it weren't for Annmarie's off-the-wall suggestion to get an RV and go out on the road. I'm looking forward to sharing the long life the information in this book points us toward.

Our growing family: Hudson Cole, Basil Rose, Jonny 5 (our cat), B (my brother's cat who rents the other litter box from us), Big Red (our lone chicken). Each of you has played a role in lightening the weight of—and at times delaying—this book writing journey.

My mom who, among many things, helped me make the decision to go back to grad school for writing. And yes, even though I didn't finish my master's degree and you're still nagging me about it, the education was essential to writing all these pages. I also thank my brother Mark, my father, and my stepfather, David, who provided inspiration from here on Earth and beyond.

My non-blood brothers: Nick Ortner for telling me years ago that *poet* and *open-mic host* were difficult career paths and for being willing to support me in just about everything I've done since college. Nick Polizzi for providing much-needed relief from writing by being my culinary teammate for joint family meals and for evenings at Revival, Jupiter, et al. Your names are only in this order because O comes before P. You guys can argue over who's number one. Gifts may help put one of you on top.

My book writing team: Lisa Miller, for keeping me on schedule in your superhuman organizational way. Autumn Millhouse, my book coach, for cheering me through the process and taking on more when I needed it. Jason Fitzroy Jeffers for handling much of the research needed to get the facts right, as well as believing in the book from the beginning. Colleen Story for your articles and research, and Diane Peters for your steady stream of on-time and almost-perfect transcription. This book would still be a Google Doc if it weren't for you five. Also to Michelle Polizzi for the seriously dangerous book cover.

The Annmarie Skin Care team, particularly Rachel Pachivas, for keeping the wheels on the bus while I was missing for days on end.

James Williams, for your constant mentorship and friendship, and most notably for loosening me up enough to enjoy my own health journey. Also our extended Peruvian family—Sebastian, Philippa, Nico, and Violeta—for your heartfelt hospitality.

The Hay House team: Reid Tracy for having faith in a grad school dropout. Patty Gift for helping me flesh out the concept and gracefully accepting my sudden pivots along the way. Laura Gray for all the brainstorming and the first round of edits, and Joan Duncan Oliver for being a badass and cutting the manuscript down from 108,000 words to 70,000 while keeping the integrity and energy of the book completely intact. You all made the book better than I could have made it alone—and gave me a 38,000-word head start on my next one.

The Renegade Health team: Frederic Patenaude for taking the reins while I was jumping from coffeehouse to coffeehouse, to write the book away from the distractions at the office, and for helping me research and brainstorm many of the concepts. Jonathan Kraft for your friendship and assistance, and Sara Murray for help taking care of all the Renegade Health customers. Gaurav Malhotra and Suzanne Rex for your help over the years.

All the experts and contributors who gave me some of their precious time, as well as those who didn't make the massive manuscript downsizing: Danny Dreyer, Daniel Vitalis, Mary Story, Heather Dane, Dede Henry, Brianna Goldstein, Frank Lucido, Mitchell Stevko, and Virgil. Special thanks to Sara Gottfried and Chris Kresser for your contributions and for your friendship and support at our monthly mindshare meetings.

# ABOUT THE AUTHOR

Kevin Gianni started seriously researching personal and preventative natural health therapies in 2002, when he was struck with the realization that cancer ran deep in his family and if he didn't change the way he was living, he might go down that same path. Since then, he has written and self-published six books on natural health, diet, and fitness; produced over 900 YouTube videos with more than 10 million views; and published hundreds of articles. Along the way, he has experimented with a wide range of diets and medical protocols in his quest to differentiate myth from reality.

Kevin has traveled all over the world searching for the best methods, foods, medicines, and clinics to introduce to readers of his blog. One of the most widely read natural health blogs on the Internet, Renegade Health (www.RenegadeHealth.com) draws hundreds of thousands of visitors a month from some 150 countries around the world. You can also follow his work at www.KevinGianni.com.

Kevin is also the co-founder, with his wife, Annmarie, of Annmarie Skin Care, a line of natural organic beauty products.

# Hay House Titles of Related Interest

YOU CAN HEAL YOUR LIFE, the movie, starring Louise Hay & Friends
(available as a 1-DVD program and an expanded 2-DVD set)
Watch the trailer at: www.LouiseHayMovie.com

THE SHIFT, the movie,
starring Dr. Wayne W. Dyer
(available as a 1-DVD program and an expanded 2-DVD set)
Watch the trailer at: www.DyerMovie.com

■ ■ ■

CRAZY SEXY KITCHEN: 150 Plant-Empowered Recipes to Ignite
a Mouthwatering Revolution, by Kris Carr

MAKE YOUR OWN RULES DIET, by Tara Stiles

THE POWER OF NO: Because One Little Word Can Bring Health, Abundance,
and Happiness, by James Altucher and Claudia Azula Altucher

THE REAL FOOD REVOLUTION: Healthy Eating, Green Groceries,
and the Return of the American Family Farm, by Congressman Tim Ryan

THE TAPPING SOLUTION: A Revolutionary System for Stress-Free Living,
by Nick Ortner

All of the above are available at your local bookstore,
or may be ordered by contacting Hay House (see next page).

■ ■ ■

We hope you enjoyed this Hay House book. If you'd like to receive our online catalog featuring additional information on Hay House books and products, or if you'd like to find out more about the Hay Foundation, please contact:

Hay House, Inc., P.O. Box 5100, Carlsbad, CA 92018-5100
(760) 431-7695 or (800) 654-5126
(760) 431-6948 (fax) or (800) 650-5115 (fax)
www.hayhouse.com® • www.hayfoundation.org

■ ■ ■

*Published and distributed in Australia by:*
Hay House Australia Pty. Ltd., 18/36 Ralph St., Alexandria NSW 2015
*Phone:* 612-9669-4299 • *Fax:* 612-9669-4144 • www.hayhouse.com.au

*Published and distributed in the United Kingdom by:*
Hay House UK, Ltd., Astley House, 33 Notting Hill Gate, London W11 3JQ
*Phone:* 44-20-3675-2450 • *Fax:* 44-20-3675-2451 • www.hayhouse.co.uk

*Published and distributed in the Republic of South Africa by:*
Hay House SA (Pty), Ltd., P.O. Box 990, Witkoppen 2068 •
info@hayhouse.co.za

*Published in India by:* Hay House Publishers India,
Muskaan Complex, Plot No. 3, B-2, Vasant Kunj, New Delhi 110 070
*Phone:* 91-11-4176-1620 • *Fax:* 91-11-4176-1630 • www.hayhouse.co.in

*Distributed in Canada by:*
Raincoast Books, 2440 Viking Way, Richmond, B.C. V6V 1N2
*Phone:* 1-800-663-5714 • *Fax:* 1-800-565-3770 • www.raincoast.com

■ ■ ■

## Take Your Soul on a Vacation

Visit www.HealYourLife.com® to regroup, recharge, and reconnect with your own magnificence. Featuring blogs, mind-body-spirit news, and life-changing wisdom from Louise Hay and friends.

Visit www.HealYourLife.com today!

# Free e-newsletters
## from Hay House, the Ultimate Resource for Inspiration

**Be the first to know about Hay House's dollar deals, free downloads, special offers, affirmation cards, giveaways, contests, and more!**

 Get exclusive excerpts from our latest releases and videos from *Hay House Present Moments*.

 Enjoy uplifting personal stories, how-to articles, and healing advice, along with videos and empowering quotes, within *Heal Your Life*.

 Have an inspirational story to tell and a passion for writing? Sharpen your writing skills with insider tips from *Your Writing Life*.

## Sign Up Now!

*Get inspired, educate yourself, get a complimentary gift, and share the wisdom!*

## http://www.hayhouse.com/newsletters.php

**Visit www.hayhouse.com to sign up today!**

 HAY HOUSE

HAYHOUSE RADIO *radio for your soul*

HealYourLife.com

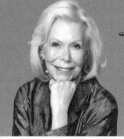
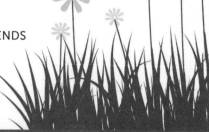